the Governor's
FOUR HEARTS

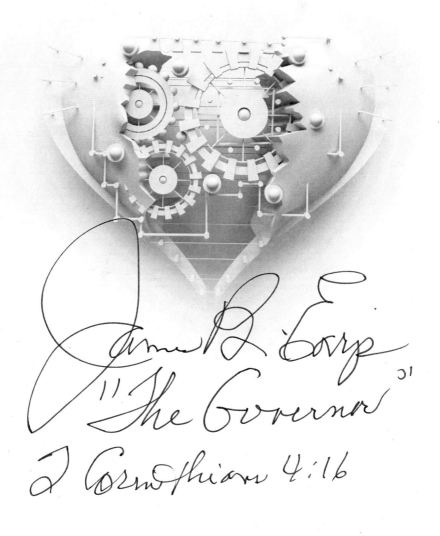

RC 2016 a good book

the Governor's
FOUR HEARTS

JAMES EARP

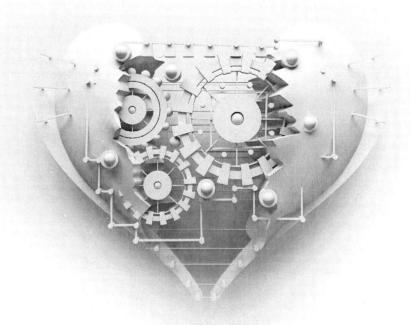

the true inspirational story of one family's
journey from death to really living

TATE PUBLISHING & *Enterprises*

Published by Tate Publishing & Enterprises, LLC
127 E. Trade Center Terrace | Mustang, Oklahoma 73064 USA
1.888.361.9473 | www.tatepublishing.com

Tate Publishing is committed to excellence in the publishing industry. The company reflects the philosophy established by the founders, based on Psalm 68:11,
"The Lord gave the word and great was the company of those who published it."

Book design copyright © 2010 by Tate Publishing, LLC. All rights reserved.
Cover design by Amber Gulilat
Interior design by Stephanie Woloszyn

Published in the United States of America

ISBN: 978-1-61739-258-0
1. Biography & Autobiography / Personal Memoirs
2. Biography & Autobiography / General
10.09.29

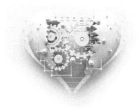

DEDICATION

This book is dedicated to my sweet family: my wife Mary, my children David Earp (deceased, 1969 -2006), and Rachel Earp Knowles, and their families, DLynn and Tatum Earp, and Clint, A.J., and Sadie Knowles, my siblings on the "front row" (This is what we came to call my brother and sisters and their spouses)–Wes and Wynelle Earp, Jo and Jack Boggs (deceased, 1936 -2006), and Molly and Bill Stringer. And finally, to my Heavenly Father without whose mercy and grace this story would not have been written.

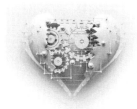

ACKNOWLEDGMENTS

I had no idea when I began to write this book what an immense undertaking it was. Along the journey to a completed manuscript from the initial ideas five years ago, a host of people have made contributions of different kinds. Some were instrumental in the first stages of determining how to begin. Some helped in the initial process to produce some audio portions of the story called "Stories from the Storm." Others did basic text entry, reading, editing, and reviewing. Some contributed greatly in clarifying details, dates, and events. Some helped in the end to make what seemed like a good manuscript even better. I am so very thankful to all those who contributed, especially to Jack and Jo Boggs, Sandy Butler, Joe Colavito, Dr. Wesley Earp, Mark Herbst, Rachel Earp Knowles, Dr. Garry Landreth, Nancy Graham Manning, Nancy Pannell, Molly Stringer, Dr. David Strutton, and David Wallis.

I especially acknowledge the contribution of my wife, Mary, who had the courage to convince me, when I believed the manuscript was complete, that the entire first part of the book needed to be rewritten. I also acknowledge with gratitude the encouragement from my editor, Sheridan Irick, to make valuable changes that I initially did not want to make because of "pride of

authorship." Thanks to my family and to the church family that
I am a part of for inspiration and support.

—James Bradley Earp, "Governor" of Texas

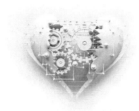

FOREWORD

"What am I holding onto? That was the question I asked James Earp on March 14, 2007 when he handed me a heavy, metal object in a hotel in Washington, D.C. You may be asking yourself a similar question about this book. So, what are you holding onto? In two words: a bridge. That's what this book offers you. James Earp opens his heart, his soul, his inner thoughts, and his family's epic story to offer you a bridge of life. Are you downcast? Do you wonder if God is really listening to you today? Are you facing what appear to be insurmountable physical or financial hurdles? Are you really living or just half-heartedly going through the motions? Whatever your current heart condition is, reading this book will strengthen your resolve to choose life, persevere, and never give up. Come along for the joyride of your life, but be prepared to journey from celebration to desperation and back again. This is not a book you read. It's a book that reads you, a story you participate in from "the front row." You will experience the full range of human emotions, from joy to grief. You will laugh. You will spill some tears. But in the end, you will realize you are holding onto authentic hope, the bridge that will lead you from faith to love. "And now these three remain: faith, hope and love. But the greatest of these is love" (1 Cor 13:13). You will love this book. It will touch your heart deeply, renew your spirit, and remind you of God's sovereign provision of mercy and grace. Read it slowly. Savor it. Let it sink in and The Governor will show you the way to really live and to really love your family, regardless of your current circumstances.

—Joe Colavito, author of *Job Track to Joyride*

" I loved my job as outpatient dietitian at the hospital. I always felt like "my" patients were like Christmas presents waiting to be unwrapped, blessings that unfolded over our visits. As it turned out, James and Mary Earp were two of my best gifts. I hadn't talked with James prior to our scheduled meeting. I only knew he was a middle-aged man who needed to lose weight.

When I entered the small waiting room, I encountered a very large, very tired, and very sad man and his wife surrounded by an unusual, repetitive, and consistent *swiiish-phoo, swiiish-phoo* sound. After introductions, I asked, "James, what is that noise?" His response was simple. "That's my heart pump." Thus began my unique relationship with Mary and James Earp.

To effectively help James, I had to have some background information about the penetrating sadness that held both Mary and James. They were obviously fairly comfortable with the LVAD and the idea that James must lose weight before a heart transplant was an option. That was certainly enough to cause grief and despair, but their pain appeared much deeper than that, more hurtful. Every patient has his own story, but I was shocked to hear James had lost his natural heart a year ago, had buried their only young son just weeks before this visit, and now needed to lose eighty pounds to be able to fit on the operating table. I soon learned that wasn't nearly their entire story.

Filling in food intake records, daily monitoring all the foods you eat, consciously counting and restricting calories for each meal and snack, and choosing only foods low in sodium are never fun things. We couldn't add exercise to James's routine because neither his heart nor his knees could handle the stress. Weight loss had to be all calorie monitoring. It is work, it is boring, it is frustrating, and it is easy to ignore, but James never did. Mary was right there with him, helping as he moved into this new eating pattern. He brought in volumes of completed food intake record sheets every visit for the next year and a half or so. His weight began to drop. In a little more than half a year, he had reached his weight goal set by his cardiologist.

Now he waited. It would be my privilege to follow many of the triumphs and the heartbreaks, the celebrations and the fears that James and Mary encountered over the next four years. James did get his fourth heart. He is still a big man, but the penetrating sadness is gone. He and Mary continue to celebrate life as he continues to maintain his health.

—Dee Rollins, PhD., R.D., L.D.

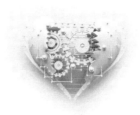

PREFACE

I did not become the "Governor of Texas" by an election. The title came during a life-threatening twenty-four day hospital stay that included nine days in ICU. I was on a ventilator. I had a morphine pump that I squeezed often for pain. My family was allowed to visit me briefly at certain time intervals. Since I was on a ventilator and could not talk, my only means of communicating with them was a pad of paper and a pencil. My sister, Jo Boggs, visited me early one morning and I signaled to her that I wanted to write her a note. She handed me the pad of paper and I scribbled, "Sister, I am going to be the Governor of Texas!" She looked at me with surprise and laughed. Since that moment, to the delight and amusement of many family and friends, I have been "The Governor."

With the morphine pump and a condition known as "ICU psychosis," I lived in an imaginary world that was vividly real to me for the nine days. In this world, I thought the nurses in ICU were plotting to kill me, so during one visit by my wife Mary, I scribbled, "They are trying to kill me in here. Take this note with you and destroy it, because I don't want them to know that I know they are trying to kill me."

But the most vivid "memory" of my time in ICU was my election campaign for Governor of Texas. My campaign slogan was "James Bradley Earp of Denton for Governor of Texas." My supporters were the small-town folk like those where I had grown up in west Texas. My campaign rallies were at roadside parks where my supporters would park their campers, lower the tailgates, and griddle waffles. This was my primary fundraiser.

Eventually in those short nine days of imaginary life, I did become Governor, but, alas, was seriously ill. My greatest disappointment was that I was supposed to address the school-children of Texas, who loved me and were gathered to hear me speak. It would be so sad and disappointing for them that I couldn't speak to them. It was at this moment that my daughter, Rachel, visited me in ICU and I scribbled to her on the notepad, "Rachel, what am I going to do about the children?" Rachel in the real world was almost nine months pregnant and would deliver her first child, A.J. Knowles, while I was still hospitalized. That morning she looked at me in utter puzzlement when I quizzed her about what we were going to do "about the children."

Then I remember vividly that in my terminal illness as Governor, a renowned Mexican physician was flown in to see if he could help. He couldn't. I was still alive and hanging on as the Governor when the real world returned, I was removed from the ventilator, and finally was moved from ICU to a room on the "heart floor," the tenth floor of Roberts Hospital on the Baylor campus. It took several days in the real world for me to begin to realize that my very vivid life had not been real at all.

Six months later, we were back at Baylor one day for a follow-up appointment and my wife, Mary, coaxed me into going back to the ICU floor just for "the memories." The first person we encountered was a nurse who immediately recognized me and hugged me. I honestly did not know how to respond to her, for in my imaginary world, she had been the very nurse who was leading the effort to kill me! Mary walked me back to the last bed in ICU where I had spent the nine days as Governor. As we stood at that point, we noticed that directly opposite my bed was the ICU break room, where it turns out that often in the morning when the shift changed, someone would use the microwave to warm up their waffles. Even as we stood there, the aroma of the waffles at the roadside park campaign fundraisers came back to me. Welcome home, Governor!

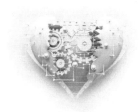

INTRODUCTION

"L ... V ... A ... D" That was the subject of literature I was reading on this desperate day, January 7, 2005. I was soon to be fifty-nine years old and wondered how much longer I would live. I had returned with the literature after a long session with Dr. Johannes Kuiper at HeartPlace at Baylor Medical Center in Dallas, Texas to my home in Denton, which was about forty miles north.

I had seen Dr. Kuiper for the first time today. Only eight days ago I had suddenly and unexpectedly almost died. I arose early on December 31, 2004, and went to the kitchen. The next thing I knew, I was coming to, collapsed on the floor amidst debris and splinters. As I lay there, I realized I had blacked out and as I fell, I crashed into the pantry and onto our granddaughter's highchair, which was now in tiny pieces surrounding me. Only a month earlier Dr. Kevin Wheelan from HeartPlace had installed an ICD/Defibrillator in my chest because of the concern my heart might stop. Thankfully, as I lay among the debris on this quiet morning, I realized the little device in my chest had done its job, shocking my heart and causing it to begin beating again. The data recorded in the device showed my heart stopped for twelve seconds!

Now as we drove back home, my wife, Mary, and I began reflecting on our session with Dr. Kuiper. Dr. Kuiper was a short, bespeckled man, and was young, surely still in his thirties. Although I had been a patient at HeartPlace at Baylor Medical center for fifteen years, this was the first time I had met with him. He is a cardiologist who primarily treats heart failure patients. My heart capacity was decreasing at an alarming rate; he would be the specialist to help me during this time. In just three months, my heart capacity would decrease below 5 percent! Today he had asked directly and boldly what I thought about an artificial heart. I told him I didn't know what to think. He urged me to take the information about the LVAD home and read it.

The literature described the "artificial heart" as a mechanical pump called a *left ventricular assist device*–thus LVAD. It was something I had never heard of in all my years as a heart patient. The statistics about the LVAD were dismal. A chapter I read became engraved in my mind. Of the people who had been implanted with an LVAD, two years later only 25 percent were still alive! It might be my only option to extend my life, but the technical information and the statistics sounded pessimistic.

Our family had already been through much sorrow and turmoil since our son David was diagnosed with Hodgkin's disease in 2001. David's treatment during the following years included six kinds of chemotherapy, three rounds of radiation, including total body radiation, and two stem cell transplants. He survived when it seemed that he might not, but with many lingering and challenging after effects of the treatment. The disease called "Graft vs. Host Disease" ravaged his body, primarily attacking his skin.

David's many hospitalizations and treatments took their toll on all of our family. We had gone through several holiday seasons darkened by his severe medical problems. As Mary and I reflected during our drive home, we had just gone through a holiday season darkened by my own severe medical problems. I did not see how any of us were up to dealing with my rapidly deteriorating heart. We had gone through too much, and I didn't want my family to go through any more.

The LVAD loomed as a last hope that might enable me to continue to live. We learned the LVAD was considered a "bridge," meaning it bought time, bridging the gap while we waited on the only real, long-term solution for heart failure: a heart transplant. Yet from our conversation with Dr. Kuiper, we knew there were some issues for me (especially my size) that might forever limit my chances for a heart transplant. It did not appear, from our conversation with him and from reading the literature, that the LVAD had ever been used as an "end therapy," a long-term solution in and of itself.

So, if I realistically had no chance for a heart transplant, what would be the use of going through all that turmoil? If the LVAD was only a bridge to a place that I would never be able to go, what was the point? I settled into a very depressing and thoughtful time. Clearly it seemed I might not live very long, even if I had the LVAD. So, as at other points in my life, I was at a crossroads. But this seemed to be the ultimate crossroads. I had lived long enough to know there would always be new challenges, and had often had to look into my own soul to see if I was up to the challenge.

This book is the story of my life and about how I came to that life-threatening point, then from that point, how I came to have *four hearts*. My purpose is that my story might be useful and inspirational in the lives of a variety of readers. This is a long journey that I am on and there have been many stations along the way. As you read this book, you are in the midst of your journey. If you are not really sure about God at all, this book is for you. If you are pretty sure about God, but you're angry or discouraged at the trouble He has allowed, this book is for you. If you are pretty sure about God and things are going well for you, but someone you know is struggling in the midst of trouble and needing help, this book is for you. If things are going well for you and all those you know, you are a blessed person, and this book is not for you. However, if you are that person, I would suggest you put the book on the shelf. There may come a time in your life when it will be for you.

SECTION 1

LIVING WITH HEART #1

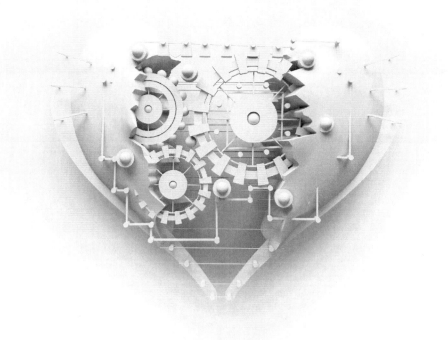

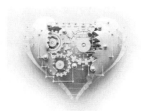

THE FORMATION OF
MY NATURAL HEART

The sand storm that was blowing was relentless. West Texas sandstorms can be frightening. The sky is darkened by the blowing sand, and it can seem like night in the middle of the day. The grit of the sand blown by winds that can gust to sixty miles an hour has a terrific blasting effect. It can blast the paint off a vehicle quickly. The grit of the sand in the mouth is an awful, distasteful effect. The sand collects into drifts just like snow and can block a road or a railroad track. The storm that occurred on March 17, 1946, was such a storm. Opal Earp gave birth that day to a ten-pound baby boy in a small hospital in Brownfield, Texas. Brownfield is aptly named. The surrounding brown landscape blends with the sand blowing in a sand storm in such a way that the horizon is not discernable.

The ten pound baby boy was me, James Bradley Earp, the future "Governor of Texas." I was not born with a silver spoon in my mouth. I was born with grit in my life. My parents, Joe and Opal Earp, had been the pioneers in their family. They moved to the plains a few years before, believing that it would be a better place to bring up their family. They farmed 320 acres of land owned by Clarence and Ima Lewis. Our house on the land had two bedrooms, but it did not have an indoor bathroom. The addition of a bathroom and bedroom to the house was an exciting time for our family when I was four years old. Our life as a family was defined by the blowing sand storms near Brownfield. It was full of sand and brown was the prominent landscape color. It was reflective of our family history. Some defining events long before I had been born made this so.

My mother's father, Jess Moore, died when she was only seven years old. One afternoon late in her life, she quietly told me of the fear and sadness she had felt, sitting alone on the front pew of the church at her father's funeral service. Her mother had been too overwhelmed with sadness and illness to attend, and her sisters were too young. She wondered in her seven-year-old mind what would happen to her mother and her sisters. Years later, at age sixteen, she married Joe Earp.

Then, in the waning days of the Great Depression, my father Joe and his cousin, Paul Cauley, had caught a life-threatening case of tularemia, or "Rabbit Fever," on a fishing trip. My father ended up in the hospital in Breckenridge, Texas where he wavered in and out of consciousness. Although he did recover, he suffered some physical and emotional effects in his life that left him aloof and private. My mother, who saw him through this near-death experience, buffered and protected him from the rest of our family all our lives. I observed later that my parents were like the velvet-covered brick. My mother was the velvet that covered the sharp edges of the brick and gave the soft covering that was needed.

Our father was a committed provider, working in the fields, pulling cotton, and working a graveyard shift at a carbon black plant when he couldn't plant a crop. In his retired years, he worked as a "grader" in the cotton-grading office. I discovered, after he died and I dealt with Mother's tax situation, that the most he earned in any one year in his life was $6,600. When he died, he did not owe anyone any money and left Opal with enough to live on comfortably in her remaining years. Yet with Opal at his side, our family was fed, clothed, and sheltered.

This largely had to do with her grit, her attitude. This was not the smooth-flowing, "Norman Vincent Peale power of positive thinking." It was toughness in the core of life that fought through the most challenging of issues and times. My mother planted that substantial grit in my life. She had come through losing her father at age seven and almost losing her husband when she had small children and was in the shadow of the Great Depression. During my time as a child in the family, she moved our family to live in four tenant farm houses, none of which people would want to raise a family in. Sand in the sand storms sifted under the window sills and door facings. She swept the sand and then mopped the floors. She planted and raised a garden and cared for farm animals that were food for our table. She found ways to encourage her husband, fix the houses up, work in the church, make clothes for our growing family, and have a meal on three times a day.

Family would come to pay us a visit from several hours away. My mother would be out the back door with our dog Alec. She would point a couple of chickens out to Alec, who would retrieve them. She would quickly wring their necks and have them plucked and ready for one of her well-known "fried chicken suppers." While Mother was working on supper, some of the cousins would gather down in the pasture to listen to Uncle Jim Jackson tell stories. I remember my cousins, Jack and David Earl Whitten, coaxing Uncle Jim into let them have a chew of his beechnut chewing tobacco. The chicken that night was delicious, but the two cousins were green around the gills, too sick to eat the delicious meal. Somehow in the sand and wind and brown, and the moving around, Opal Earp lived a "gritty, can-do" kind of life. She denied herself and helped others. She encouraged me. Throughout my life, I have been blessed with her "Yes, it can be done." God cares, and He will show up in His time if one walks by faith! It became entirely possible that a ten-pound baby boy, born in poverty during a sandstorm in Brownfield, Texas, on St. Patrick's Day would one day be the Governor of Texas!

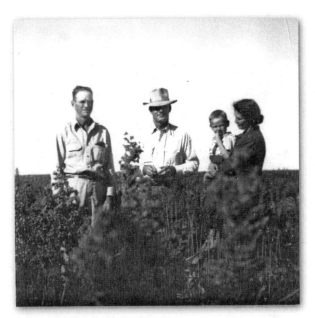

The 3 year old Governor with his parents and Uncle Jim

I am the youngest of four children. My brother Wes is fourteen and a half years older than me, and we have two sisters: Jo, who is nine years older than me, and then Molly, who is six years older than me. Our family farmed tenant farms owned by others. There were several occasions in my growing up when my family moved due to ownership changes of the land. During my elementary school years, I attended four different schools. One of those schools was a small, rural, two-room school named, amazingly, "Sandhill School" in a little village named "Sandhill" that had one school, one store, and two churches in Floyd County on the high plains of Texas. I was born in Brownfield and was educated in Sandhill. The fourth, fifth, and sixth grades were all in one room with one teacher. This unusual environment enabled me to complete three grades in two years!

Family was the heart issue in my development as a child. In the rural areas where we lived there was hot weather, dust, and not much excitement. We did get a daily newspaper, *The Ft. Worth Star Telegram*, which came a day late through the mail. I read the paper as soon as I was able to read, and before I could read, someone in my family read the comics to me. Our family attended church regularly and music, both at church and at home, was a big part of our life. We had a piano and both my sisters learned to play.

By the time I was four years old, I developed an early interest in and passion for baseball that continues to this day. We lived about twenty miles from Lamesa, Texas, which had a minor league professional baseball team named the Lamesa Lobos. I have fond memories of going with my parents and my brother, Wes, to Lamesa to see the Lobos play. Many farmers watched from behind the wire backstop, waiting for "T-Bone" Miller to come to the plate. He often hit long home runs, and after he trotted around the bases, he would run along the backstop where the farmers would put rolled-up dollar bills through the wire. He would gather a handful before he went back to the bench. He was the big reason Lamesa, in 1950, was known as the biggest little city in professional baseball. The Lobos had a total attendance that summer of more than 100,000 fans. One night "T-Bone" collected $149 after hitting several home runs. The next morning, he approached team management and demanded a $100 bonus, insisting the reason the fans came out was to watch him hit home runs. The bonus was quickly paid.

My older brother, Wes, cast a giant shadow of a role model in my life.

He was a solid "six-footer," and by the time I was fourteen years old, I had grown to 6'2" and weighed over 200 pounds. Joe Earp enjoyed telling people that he and Opal didn't have boys; they had a couple of strong mules!

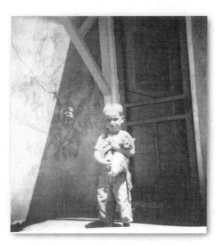

Governor holds his kitty and waits for Wes to take him on a date

I rode the school bus with my sisters. We were always vulnerable to the weather, especially the sand storms, as that was a time of great drought in our part of Texas. The strong winds blew the sand into drifts that the school bus got stuck in. Its seems scary to me now as I remember a dark day when the bus got stuck and the driver left the bus to walk through the blowing sand to a farm about a mile away to get a farmer to bring his tractor and pull the bus through the sand.

The little stucco house where we lived was not very tight around the windows, so in the midst of the sandstorms, there was always an accumulation of dust on the window sills. Art supplies were unknown to us, so I would use my fingers to draw pictures and practice my printing on all the windowsills in the house!

Our family took some adventurous trips, with other extended family traveling along with us. We had a tarp top that fit over the bed of our 1950 Ford pickup, and we traveled to various places in New Mexico to sightsee and fish ... places like Cloudcroft, the "White Sands," Ruidoso, some favorite fishing places along the Rio Grande River, and Red River. Some slept outdoors on cots, and some slept in the back of the pickup. Meals cooked over a campfire were a memorable part of those trips. Such adventures were big fun and built relationships with our extended family. Observers would have surely deemed us poor, but I never really felt that way.

But by the year 1953, surely we were poor. The drought was so severe that my father was unable to plant a crop! We did have some advantages in that we lived on a farm and had some cows for milk, and we had pigs and chickens for eggs and meat. Our mother was a master at feeding a hungry family, coaxing the garden to grow peas, corn, okra, watermelon, and cantaloupe. Two events about her and her formidable "grit" from my childhood are burned in my mind, never to be forgotten.

One day it was very hot. My mother drove to where she was going to hoe the weeds from the garden. Even though it was dry, "careless" weeds and "white" weeds were notorious in their ability to thrive in the dry heat. As she got out of our old Frazier car that day, my mother took her hoe and dug a large hole near the base of the largest "careless" weed around. Then she had me sit in the hole in the shade of the "careless" weed to keep me cool. Later, I would read and memorize the scripture from Psalms 91 that talks about a mighty eternal shade and says, "He who dwells in the shelter of the Most High will rest in the shadow of the Almighty. I will say of the Lord. 'He is my refuge, and my fortress, my God in whom I trust.'" From my earliest meditations on that verse, I have in my mind the shade that my mother Opal made for me that day.

Her garden "shelter" was more vivid and dangerous on another day. That day, she arrived in the morning to pick some vegetables to cook for the family's lunch. When she got out of the old Frazier, she told me to play in the turn row beside the garden while she picked the vegetables that were ready. She was such a soft and gentle person, but in a moment she appeared out of the garden very agitated and quickly opened the trunk of the car and got the tire changing tools from inside. Then she turned and looked very sharply into my eyes and said, "Sonny, do not move from this place!" She quickly took the tire tools into the garden. In a few minutes she came out of the garden with the tire tools and with her sacks of vegetables to cook for lunch. She loaded the items in the trunk and we got into the car and went to the house. Only later did I come to know that on that morning, with me playing on the turn row, she had been picking okra. When she came to the tallest okra stalk, she was frightened by a diamondback rattlesnake coiled around the okra stalk. Without a word spoken, she had hurried back and gotten the tire tool, killed the rattlesnake, finished gathering the vegetables, and returned to the car. She had fixed lunch and fed the family, all before anyone knew about the rattlesnake. Her "shade" would loom big in my life later when other fearful, life-threatening times came to me. As God would whisper quietly in my thought-life years later, I could hear her gritty, "can-do" whisper in concert with His voice.

Finally in the fall of 1953, with no harvest and not much prospect for the future, it was time for a big change. My aunt and uncle, Nellie and E.A. McBeth, lived on an irrigated farm near Kress, Texas, further up on the plains. What our family needed was an irrigated farm to avoid the calamity of the drought. My uncle E.A. had a noticeable limp and had to have help with his farming. My parents had lived with this aunt and uncle back in Haskell County when they first married and my father did the farming for Uncle Ezra. At this strategic crossroads in our family's life, they returned the favor. So we moved in with them into their two-bedroom farmhouse, my sisters and I sleeping on the living room floor.

I was a second grader. The difficulty and challenge of the time escaped me as it seemed to me we were on a perpetual living room campout at their house. They had a television! I enjoyed eating ice cream and lying on the carpet, watching *Six Gun Theatre*. Oblivious to me was the fact that my parents pulled cotton in the fields every day that fall to make enough money to survive. Before Christmas, the deal was concluded to have them become the renters of an irrigated 160 acre farm about a mile from my aunt's and uncle's. We returned to our old place at Wellman on a weekend and used the car, pickup, trailers, and tractor to bring all our belongings to live on the new place. It had a very small house with a living room, a bedroom for my parents, and a combination room where my sisters and I slept and where our kitchen table was located adjacent to a very small kitchen. I went to the second grade and part of the third at Kress Elementary School, riding the school bus about eight miles into town.

As the years passed, we lived near Kress and then Floydada, Texas. My siblings all married and for several years, I was alone at home with my parents.

My earliest memories include a favorite dog, "Alec," who chased cars that passed our house on the dirt country roads where we lived. When my family lived near Floydada and I went to school at Sandhill School, one side of our farm was bordered by a black top highway. One hot July morning I experienced my greatest childhood loss. We were hoeing cotton near the highway and Alec was with us. He began to chase a car that was passing by on the highway and he didn't see a car coming from the opposite direction. The driver was not able to avoid hitting Alec, who had chased his last car. I was so sad over the loss of this dear pet.

As I reflect now with my fourth heart, this memory reminds me of the reading that I have done about the history of open-heart surgery as pioneered by Dr. Walt Lillihi and others, many of them associated with the University of Minnesota. Their early tests in the 1940s and early 1950s were done in the laboratory using dogs. Because dog hearts have similarities to human hearts, the doctors used them in their first experimental surgeries. The dogs' lives were sacrificed as early experience was gained with open-heart surgery. So, a heart transplant not only requires the loss of life of a donor, but in the years of perfecting heart surgery, it involved the loss of the lives of many laboratory dogs.

In my seventh grade year, we moved to Munday, Texas, where I would eventually graduate from high school. During these years, I was the only child left at home. I was quiet and often alone and I have good memories of walking through the wheat fields at night under a starlit sky, dreaming about the future. Actually, I was a dreamer, often imagining myself in some heroic role while I was really just hoeing cotton.

I grew up with a strong work ethic, but I gradually came to the conclusion that I did not want to spend my adult life on a farm. My brother, Wes, had blazed a trail as an educator, becoming the first in our large extended family to earn a doctorate degree. Wes was a good role model for me. I was a very good student, so a good education seemed to be the way to avoid being a farmer.

So it was as I endured "senioritis" as a senior at Munday High School, a few weeks from graduation.

Life growing up on a farm near a small town had its advantages, and grace was abundant as God, through my parents, teachers, and principals, led me, no matter how unaware I was of his leading. This spring "senioritis" day, my parents were planning to go fishing after I left on the school bus. I pleaded with them to let me skip school and go along, and they agreed! It was a great day, until the next morning, when I realized that I would have to take a written excuse to school for my absence the previous day. I certainly didn't want to jeopardize my upcoming graduation. I told my mother I needed an excuse, and I remember well as she sat down and wrote out an honest excuse. "Mr. Knudson, please excuse my son, James Earp, for missing class yesterday. He went fishing with his dad and me. We had a good time, Opal Earp."

Mr. Knudson was in only his first year as principal of Munday High School, but he was a veteran teacher and had been a principal in several other school districts. I went into his office and gave him my excuse. He had surely seen every excuse in the book. He read it and laughed and said, "Get on back to class son!" A few days later, one of my teachers told me that Mr. Knudson wanted to see me in his office. After I entered, he walked over and closed the door. What an ominous moment! I didn't know what to say, or what I had done wrong. He sat down. He looked at me with his dark eyes, which seemed capable of penetrating the hardest metal. Then he said to me, to the best of my memory, "Son, I am going to tell you something today that I am not supposed to, but I am going to, anyway. Your IQ score is the highest of any student that has ever been recorded in this county. The seniors are about to graduate and most of them have no idea about what they are going to do with their lives. They may try college, or follow in their families footsteps, living on the farm and raising a family. But you are different. You have been given a great gift. Son, I want you to promise me that you will do something with your life, because you have been blessed with the ability to do much." That was such an unexpected crossroads moment that shaped and continues to challenge me, even to this very day.

I grew up going to small Baptist churches and had a heritage of faith. I was younger than my peers and wished to "fit in" so I had some adolescent experiences of sowing "wild oats," which, in the culture that I grew up, in meant drinking beer on the sly in a dry county, driving too fast, and staying out too late. I concealed the kind of seed that I was sowing, still sitting by my mother at church on Sunday mornings. I did realize the hypocrisy of not especially living a lifestyle that was reflective of our Christian beliefs.

I took that same lifestyle into my early college years where, to support myself, I worked for a local manufacturing company loading trucks. It was hard work, but after the rigors of growing up on the farm, I was well prepared. I often worked late into the night and then attended early morning classes. My language reflected the sweaty truck-loading culture where I spent many hours. I remember one night the dock manager saying to me, "Earp, you have the dirtiest mouth I have ever heard!" I was only eighteen years old and I had already achieved much: a foul mouth that was beyond compare in his eyes.

Within the first three semesters of school, I tired of the bad reputation and worked to turn over a new leaf and find a new connection with church and with the fellowship of students at the Baptist Student Union.

Mary Graham and I met as students at the University of North Texas in Denton, Texas. We met in the fellowship of the Baptist students at UNT. Mary was a Home Economics major.

I had first attended college at Texas A&M, but I transferred to UNT, where eventually I got a Bachelor of Arts in English. I took many math classes. Mary came from a family in Collingsworth County. She had an older brother and younger sister. I had dated other girls at UNT, but Mary is the one I was continually drawn to.

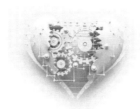

MY NATURAL HEART CHANGES

Whether by habit or family expectation, I always made it to church on Sunday morning. As time went by, I became dissatisfied with the way I had lived in my early college days. I cannot recall the specific moment this happened. Perhaps it was actually a thought process that brought me to that conclusion. I was inspired to intensify my involvement in church and Christian student life. I determined to finish my degree so I could move on to the fulfillment of some of my childhood dreams. By perspiration and inspiration, I completed my college degree in three years, graduating at age twenty.

Somehow, even with finishing the degree in three years and working hard loading trucks, I spent time at the Baptist Student Union on campus. I would hang out and play Ping-Pong or "42" and along the way, I got to know lots of students. Of course, the one student that I really wanted to know well was Mary Graham. I would sit and read the newspaper and stare at her sitting and studying in a chair across the room. As I think back on it now, I am not so sure she was studying. She may have been a crafty girl herself, as she sat and smiled at me and batted her eyelashes. However, she was not in the "42" or Ping-Pong clique, so it took me a while to ask her out. We both had leadership roles in the BSU, so we were naturally around one another for planning meetings.

I was game for about anything that came along. I was asked by a couple of guys at the BSU to go along one Sunday afternoon and observe as they conducted a Bible study at the Denton County jail. This was out of my "comfort zone," but I agreed to go along and observe. I dressed in my only suit and tie and found my biggest Bible to take with me. When I arrived at the Denton County jail, neither of my friends was there. I lingered for a little while, waiting for them to show up. It took a while for me to realize that they were not going to show up, and my anxiety level skyrocketed as it became clear that I was not just an observer, but the one and only "presenter." The jail was on the fifth floor of the building, and soon the jailer said to me, "Are you ready for me to take you up?"

I shook my head and gulped, having no preparation or awareness of what was about to happen. I wondered as we rode the elevator up how big the chapel was and if there would be many men in it. When the elevator doors opened, he led me along in front of the bars of what was apparently the main holding "tank." It was filled to capacity with men who were playing cards and blowing smoke out through the bars. Before I knew what was happening, the jailer had gone back into the elevator to go downstairs. I was alone in this frightening and hard place! I took my Bible and began to stammer and read and try to think of something pertinent to say. The men just starred at me and blew smoke in my eyes. I remember turning quickly and returning to the elevator and banging on the call button. I tried to maintain some sense of composure until the jailer arrived back on the elevator to retrieve me. Mine was surely the shortest and least impactful sermon ever preached at the Denton County jail.

On the drive back to the campus, I told myself that that was one place I would never go back to. Never say never in life.

My relationship with Mary blossomed. I now had a staff position at First Baptist Church in Denton. My position included responsibility for college students, and when Mary came back to start her senior year at UNT, I made sure to seek her out after church and ask her for her phone number! We enjoyed dating that fall and before Christmas, we seemed to know that we were meant for each other. We had one major hurdle on our way to falling in love. It involved homecoming. Mary had never had a mum for homecoming. This was her senior year, and her last chance. I planned to call her up and have that special time at the game so she could show off her mum. The system for calling in to the women's dormitories was archaic and inefficient. There was only one phone on the floor for a number of young women, and this phone was constantly busy. I tried many times to reach Mary, with no success. Finally, in desperation on the Saturday morning of the game, I drove to her dorm to try to find her. That morning she was not to be found! My frugal tendencies kicked in: it was game time and a beautiful and expensive mum was about to go to waste, so I stopped by the BSU building where there were some students gathered who did not have dates. I saw a senior girl that I knew there and impulsively gave Mary's mum to her!

This comedy of errors helped me see that I was in love with Mary. I had to do something to make amends. I made the quickest and best investment decision I have ever made. I scraped the bottom of my financial resources and ordered a beautiful box of a dozen red roses to be delivered to Mary at her dorm. By the time I saw her, she had forgiven me and it was clear that she was in love with me! Oh, how sweet it is! Soon we were making plans to be married.

Mary completed her degree that spring, and I worked up to ninety-six hours a week that summer in the same plant where I had worked on the dock, trying to save enough money so that we could have a financial head start on our marriage. Mary spent June and July back at her home on the farm preparing for our marriage. She made her own wedding dress as well as the bridesmaids' dresses. We were married at the First Baptist Church in Wellington, Texas, on August 13, 1967. Mary was twenty-two years old and I was twenty-one. I was younger than her, but I was big and no one seemed aware of any age difference.

After a week honeymooning in Colorado, we loaded a U-Haul trailer and headed for Louisville, Kentucky, where I had planned to go to Southern Baptist Theological Seminary to prepare for a career in ministry. We had no jobs, and upon our arrival, we discovered that we did not have a place to live. Our love was oblivious to all the question marks and hurdles. Almost immediately a need for Mary to have oral surgery drained our savings, and we began to wonder if we would get work and be able to pay our bills. Never fear: I was the gritty sonny-boy of Opal's. There was always a way.

After the local schools had already started, Mary was able to get a job teaching home economics at Charlestown High School in Charlestown, Indiana. She commuted with some other teachers whose husbands were also in seminary. We settled into a busy newly-married life, with going to school and becoming very involved at a local church where I had a part-time staff position. During the two years we lived in Louisville, I would also work assisting a man who painted houses, and then I took a part-time job in the hardware department of Sears.

Just remembering the job of painting houses reminds me of the most significant miracle that occurred in our early married life. I worked for a teacher who had a "moonlight" business of painting houses. After school or on Saturdays, we would meet at someone's house and my job was to do the scraping in preparation for the paint. By the time it got dark, we would clean up and head our separate ways to his home and my apartment. He had a 1957 Chevrolet station wagon that served as the "paint wagon" with all the paint and supplies in it. As we cleaned up, the tailgate of the station wagon would be down and when we were through, he would close it.

One day as I cleaned my hands, I took off my almost-new, shiny wedding ring and laid it on the tail fin of the station wagon. There was barely enough room for the ring to rest there. We finished cleaning up and I headed home. My boss lived several miles across Louisville from where we were, and he had several train tracks to cross and many busy intersections to get though before getting home. I got to our apartment long before he got home, and when I kissed Mary, she immediately noticed that my wedding ring was missing! What a loss! I called the boss's home and talked to his wife about what happened, but he had not gotten home yet. We agreed that there was not much likelihood the ring would be found, due to its precarious position and the distance and bumpiness of the ride. Later the phone rang and it was my boss, who excitedly told me that when he went back out to check, the wedding ring was still perched precariously on the tail fin! As I write this, I am looking down at that ring on my finger with the greatest sense of blessing about how God has watched over and provided for Mary and me in our marriage.

We visited our family in the summer after our first year in Louisville, and when we returned to Louisville in the fall, Mary started teaching before my seminary classes started. I began to try to find part-time work, and she found out that at her high school there was an unfilled position for a high school math teacher. Her principal asked her if I could substitute while they tried to find someone before my seminary classes started. The substitute teaching money was better than any of my previous part-time jobs. My analytical and math abilities emerged and I enjoyed the challenge of teaching math. By the time I had to register for my classes, the principal met with me and tried to convince me to continue teaching. He had not been successful in finding a permanent teacher. He assured me that he would be able to help me get an emergency Indiana teaching certificate.

Mary and I thus encountered another "crossroads moment." After careful thought and prayer, we decided that I would register for night seminary classes and continue to teach the algebra and geometry classes for the year. This brought some nice time in our young married life as we packed our lunches and drove to school together. We didn't yet realize that a new direction was emerging in our lives.

The principal encouraged us to attend a conference for teachers on a Saturday, and the focus of my math conference was a small Olivetti Underwood programmable calculator. It was my first exposure to any kind of computer-like device. My math skills had been honed in high school, as I competed in "number sense" and even had the highest technology of the day: a slide rule. I was fascinated with this first exposure to a computer. There were no curricula in computer science in those days and the computer industry was at an absolute ground floor time. Companies such as IBM, Burroughs, and Honeywell were anxious to hire people with analytical skills who could quickly get up to speed in their mushrooming need for computer programming.

By the next spring, we came to another exciting and life-changing crossroads. Mary went to the doctor and we were excited to find out that she was pregnant. We realized that if we were going to have a family, we would want to live back in Texas where we would be nearer our families. I was within fifteen hours of completing my seminary degree, but by now I was realizing that my analytical and math skills were an undeniable part of who I was. I began to believe that to support a family with a child I was being led to consider the opportunities in the computer industry. We sought counsel about the dilemma of not completing the seminary degree and a ministry career, making a change at this pivotal moment. I knew that my mother especially wanted a minister son, and I dreaded the thought of communicating to her a new direction in life outside of the ministry.

One of the aspects of my math teaching job was that I did not have an actual classroom. I floated from one room to another for each of my classes. During my preparation period, I had to use the school library. One morning I picked up a magazine in the library and flipped through it. There was a full page advertisement by IBM in Dallas, Texas, for those with a college degree who could demonstrate an aptitude to be a computer programmer. Mary and I discussed the possibility of responding to the ad, and decided that it might be divine providence that I respond. So within two weeks I was flying to Dallas for an aptitude test and an interview with IBM!

IBM had a computer software development center in Boca Raton, Florida, and because of my high aptitude score, I was offered a job there. However, Florida is a long way from Texas, so we decided not to accept the offer. But the high score and clear aptitude gave us confidence that something might open up in this field that I now seemed destined for. Soon I had an interview with Burroughs Corporation in Dallas where, again, I scored well on the aptitude test and was offered a job as a computer programmer. By July, 1969, we had pulled a trailer loaded with all our possessions back to Denton, Texas where we rented an apartment. I began a daily commute to Dallas, quickly being mentored into productivity as a programmer. We had only one car, and Mary was now very pregnant. At 6:25 each morning she drove me to the Continental Trail bus station for the bus trip to downtown Dallas. I walked ten blocks to the Burroughs offices on North Harwood Street.

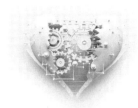

MY NATURAL HEART AS A FATHER

In August we toured Flow Hospital in Denton in preparation for the birth of our child. Dixie Clardy, a church friend who was a hospital volunteer, conducted the tour. When she found out what I was doing, she encouraged me to apply for a computer position with Moore Business Forms in Denton where her husband worked. She knew they had an opening. About this time we began the paperwork to buy a small new home, sensing that we might be destined to live in Denton a long time. The house paperwork moved quickly and the last week of August we moved into our first home, somewhat anxious about our ability to make a huge house payment of $153 per month.

Mary busied herself, getting curtains made and hung, thinking that we had until the third week of September for the baby to come. On Labor Day, September 1, I labored mightily to rake and seed grass in our new yard. On Saturday, Mary's water broke and we realized that she was going into labor herself! She began to have contractions, and we hurried to Flow Hospital. By the early morning hours of Sunday, September 7, 1969, she had given birth to our son, David Bradley Earp. He was two weeks early and weighed only six pounds and two ounces. He was healthy, however, and once we brought him home, he began to gain weight.

Meanwhile, I had an interview with Moore Business Forms for the open position. They administered the same aptitude test that I had previously done well on. Before the month was out I had been offered a job and begun work in Denton as a Systems Analyst with Moore, commencing a twenty-two year career. Our family was so blessed to have me working locally. I was even able to come home for lunch.

We were an integral part of our old church, First Baptist Church of Denton. David was enrolled on the "cradle roll." He first attended a worship service when he was six weeks old, sitting on his mother's lap on the back row. We renewed old friendships and made new ones. Within two years I would be ordained as a very young deacon.

Rachel was born on March 22, 1971 when David was only eighteen months old. We had two children in diapers. Mary was busy practicing her home economics profession at home. I advanced in my career. Along the way, we made a brief career stop at a Moore plant in Greenwood, South Carolina.

In 1980 we moved to Libertyville, Illinois, where I had been promoted to the position of National Manager of Information Systems with Moore. Less than a year later, we were back in Texas, moving into the home where we still live as I became part of a new computer focused division of Moore.

David and Rachel did well in school. They loved their life in church and had lots of friends and pets. Mary was involved in many aspects of our church and in all the kids' school activities. Life was good. Those childhood dreams of long ago seemed fulfilled. It seemed even more so as David and Rachel moved into their junior high and high school years.

In 1984 the summer Olympics were to be held in Los Angeles and for a year prior to that, we had planned a long vacation to drive to California from Denton and attend some of the

Olympic events. We drove our big, red Buick west from Texas, stopping by the Grand Canyon to sightsee. Then we moved onto Las Vegas. The place didn't appeal to any of us, so packed up and drive on to California. When we left after our one night in Vegas, on the way out of town, David pleaded to stop in front of Caesar's Palace. He wanted to go in and get a match book to add to his match book collection. I consented and drove up and parked illegally with the flashers on while the girls waited in the car. Dave and I went in to find his match book. After Dave got the match book, I decided that it was a good teaching situation for my fourteen-year-old son. So I told him I wanted him to see firsthand how quickly money could disappear in Las Vegas. I showed him a dollar I had. I changed it into four quarters and immediately put two quarters into a slot machine and pulled the handle. Nothing happened. I gave him my "I told you so" look and put the other two quarters in and pulled the handle. The most amazing thing happened: quarters started pouring out of the machine. There were so many that I had to get a large cottage cheese-like container to catch them. Was I ever embarrassed as David ran back to the car with the cottage cheese-container of quarters! He was yelling, "Mom, guess what Dad did!"

When we got into California and stopped to eat at a Taco Bell in Barstow, I paid for our lunch with quarters, and the teenager taking our order said, "I know where you have been!" So much for my lifestyle teaching moments.

One of our funniest and most memorable moments as a family occurred at this point in our trip. Our only night spent in the bay area was at a motel in Oakland. We were all excited and anticipated spending the whole day on the wharf and riding the streetcars of San Francisco. We loaded up our Buick early that morning to head out. As I backed out, I missed seeing a "high rider" pickup behind me and crunched our trunk on its big steel bumper. I got out to survey the damage. There was none to the heavy pickup bumper, but the entire trunk lid of our Buick was mashed in. I tried the key, but the trunk would not open. *What a dilemma!* Our one day to do all these exciting things and we had a trunk that would not open! We had a motel reservation the next night in Palo Alto, California. Then we were due in Los Angeles the next night for the opening Olympic event we had tickets for.

So what would we do? Being the optimistic and adventurous family that we were, we ignored the problem, went into San Francisco, and had a great day. We then found ourselves in front of the motel at Palo Alto at 11 p.m. without a way to open the trunk! David and I got the girls into the room and assured them that we would return soon, thinking there must be some way to get the trunk open. It was now almost midnight and there was nothing open, until we found a deserted all-night gas station. This was before the days of convenience stores. It was truly a gas station, with two teenaged attendants who had opposite personalities.

By then David was a husky 6 foot, 200 pound fourteen year old. He was a shadow of his dad, who was 6'4" and weighed 275 pounds. We were two big Texans. David had worn white pants that day, and had bought as a souvenir a green surgical gown-looking shirt that said on the back, "Outpatient San Francisco Psychiatric Ward." So we pulled into the station in our big Buick with Texas tags and a crunched trunk and asked the first high school boy working if he had a crowbar that we could borrow. The other high school boy coworker was obviously a cautious fellow, and when he saw us, he hurried back into the station and put his hands over his eyes and said, "I'm not watching this."

The other worker enthusiastically got into what was going on and led us back into the shop where we found a large four-foot-long metal rod. Meanwhile his cautious coworker, who had holed himself up in the office, was yelling in a loud voice, "I'm not having anything to do with this!" We took the big rod and David and I took turns hitting the car trunk lock with it. Eventually, after many licks, we were successful in punching the lock out, the trunk popped open. Ever prepared, we found a bungee cord in the trunk that would hold the trunk lid down now that the lock was gone. Ever after, even in the darkest moments of our lives, David and I would think about this night and laugh until we cried.

We did make it to all the Olympic events and had a great time. Our only downside is that we spent ten nights on the road with a trunk lid held down only by a bungee cord.

David's major project when we returned home was to restore the 1966 Chevrolet pickup that his grandfather, Joe Earp, had owned. My dad had just passed away a few months before, and his old pickup sat forlornly beside my mother's house in Knox City, Texas. It was in poor repair, and there was no more finish on the body of the pickup due to unrelenting wind and sand that were blowing in that area. David had asked his Granny Earp if he could have the pickup, and she quickly and gladly agreed.

So with the pickup back in Denton, he spent every spare moment working on it. His money came from his job, as he worked with his friends for Harry Koch, a local shop teacher and family friend. It seemed sort of a rite of passage for many teenaged boys in Denton to earn their first paychecks by slinging picks and shoveling rocks and dirt in order to make trenches for water sprinkler systems. It was hard work but David relished it, as he was gaining ground on the needed financial resources for the pickup renovation project.

Before school started, he had replaced the rotted out pickup bed and Tommy Stevens had helped him paint the pickup a beautiful Texas Aggie maroon. When he got the motor running one day, the seat wasn't back from the upholstery shop. So he convinced me that we could put two lawn chairs in the pickup and drive it. We drove down University Drive with the new stereo loudly blaring "Be Strong and Courageous!" by Michael W. Smith.

By the time we got to I-35, we were talking about how much fun it would be to drive as far north on I-35 as it is possible to go. Years later, Mary and I were driving on I-35 north though Duluth, Minnesota. I called David, who was on a photo shoot in Milwaukee at the time, and told him we were about to come to the end of I-35 in Duluth, Minnesota,

Back in Denton, ending our drive on University Drive, we came by the upholstery shop to get the completed front seat. In a few days school would start and David would have his sixteenth birthday on Monday of the week school started. This enabled a whole hoard of sophomore boys to fill the bed of the pickup on the way to lunch during the new Denton High open campus.

Moore went through some changes, and just after we had gone to the Olympics in 1984, I had the opportunity to go to work in Denton as the vice president of a small computer training company named Hypergraphics, started by Dr. Darrell Ward. He and I traveled extensively, soliciting business and new opportunity for the company. Four years later, the challenge of helping to build the cutting edge business had become a challenge to our need for financial security as David would soon be graduating from high school and going off to college.

Unexpectedly, I was offered a job back with the sales organization of Moore, covering all the states in the southern part of the country as a Regional Systems manager. I traveled constantly, making presentations to major customers in most of the large cities of the south. I carried a laptop computer and a projector with me. I was in constant motion. I was forty-four years old and had never really had a major health crisis.

Even though I traveled so much in these years, we still had a great family life. When David and Rachel were in high school, they hosted a fun "dress-up Christmas party" at our home that all the kids loved to come to. They would dress up in their finest, come to our house, stand around and talk and visit and drink punch and eat all kinds of things that we cooked. They stayed until the wee hours. On at least two of these occasions, we had more than 150 teenagers in our house at a time. It was great fun! One night the punchbowl broke and the young people continued to stand around and visit, oblivious to the fact that Mary and I were crawling around on our hands and knees, mopping up ice and punch. They never stopped talking and hardly noticed that soon a second punch bowl was in place with ice and some fresh punch. These were great times. Needless to say, we were exhausted after each of them. However, we still believe that memories are always worth what you invest in them.

Then there was the day before David's graduation from Denton High School. His career as a Denton Bronco tackle had been shortened by a bad back injury, but he seemed to always land on his feet and by his senior year, he was president of the student body. As a result, he seemed to have the run of the school with no concern about being out of class on "official business." Rachel always thought things were easy for him and he got away with too much and she was right. He charmed Mrs. Bateman, other teachers, and the staff all along the way, especially during his senior year, when he was both student body president and a National Merit Scholar. He and Rachel were in the same chemistry class, and she remembers the blessed days he had as well. I was home for lunch this day, and David was rummaging around upstairs. I asked him when he came down what he was up to, and he casually said, "Oh ... nothing, Dad."

He got in his pickup and headed back to school where his chemistry class was to start at one p.m. Unknown to any of us, David had misplaced his chemistry notebook, and was trying to find it in his room at home before his last class started and it was due. Later we would hear that as David screeched to a halt at a red light at Carroll Boulevard, he heard a thud, and he looked down to see the missing Chemistry workbook slide out from under the seat. He confidently got back to high school just in time to march in triumphantly carrying his chemistry workbook. That was so David. As a junior, he was the lead player on the Whiz Kid team that won the national finals in Columbus, Ohio. He did not compete as a senior, as he didn't want his buddies to perceive him as some kind of "geek."

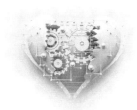

MY NATURAL HEART - DAMAGED!

The major health crisis came to me in January of 1990. I was hospitalized with severe viral pneumonia at Denton Community Hospital. My fever raged, reaching 107 degrees on the third day. Finally, the fever broke and I returned home, very weak after the ordeal. Within a month I was back to my travel, but noticed that when I stood to collect my things after a flight, my head was dizzy. The next week when I was home I went to see Dr. Jitendra Bhatt. He is an internist, one of the doctors who cared for me in my hospital stay. He did an EKG and other tests. He expressed concern that I had some kind of unusual heart problem that he did not feel equipped to diagnose.

He referred me to Dr. Kevin Wheelan at the HeartPlace at Baylor Medical Center in Dallas. In March, 1990, I was admitted to Baylor, where I spent a week being checked and tested. At the end of the week, Dr. Wheelan met with Mary and me and told us that the high fever and the viral pneumonia had damaged my heart. The resulting condition was called cardiomyopathy. We had never heard of this condition. He explained that with cardiomyopathy, over time my heart would weaken, losing its capacity to pump my blood. We were shocked when he said that this condition always leads to heart failure, a terminal illness. Then he soberly said that he believed that if I lived to be age sixty, it would be with a heart transplant. This would be the beginning of the journey that would see me have four hearts. So began a series of life challenges that covered the next nineteen years of my life.

Over time, our routine returned to normal and I was busy traveling and working again. New prescription medication took care of the dizziness, and life seemed just as it had always been. David had gone to Texas A&M as a Presidential Scholar and Rachel was at Wake Forest University in North Carolina studying Russian. We were busy trying to keep everything afloat financially. With these issues pressing, I gave very little thought to the possibility of heart failure and the grim prospect that Dr. Wheelan had given us. I did well, exercising and taking care of my health. First, I saw Dr. Wheelan every year. But as time passed and I did well, the scheduled check-ups were only every three years.

Meanwhile, business challenge was accelerating. Moore had been the industry leader my entire career, but now the impact of technology on the business forms industry began to have a serious impact on our business. There were consolidations, reorganizations, firings, and downsizings. What had been fulfilling in the past became a grind with constant pressure. Although I could not perceive the impact on my health, in retrospect, I can look back and see that the stress did much damage to the strength of my fragile natural heart.

I was in a constant travel mode, and one night in July, 1991, I picked up a voicemail when I was in Kansas City from my boss, Travis McWhorter. Only six months before, in the midst of some difficult personnel cutbacks, I had posed the question of what would happen to our careers to Travis. He had laughed it off, saying, "you are so well thought-of within the company. If something happens, you will be the last guy out, turning the lights out!"

The voicemail from Travis had asked that I meet him at the Admirals Club at DFW Airport when I flew in the next day. I realized as I sat in my hotel room that night that my career with Moore was over. I prayed and pleaded with God, explaining to Him the pressure of having our two kids in college and the unfairness of this happening to a long-term loyal employee. I was forty-five years old and not ready for this. My thoughts were not just musing about what would happen. In my heart, I *knew* what would happen the next day. I had just had to do the same to other loyal, long-term employees only months before. Somehow God gave me grace, and I arrived at the ominous meeting the next day, hanging onto my composure. It was exactly as I had thought. As it turns out, I was not the last to leave, turning off the lights when I left. A senior executive had flown halfway across the country to tell me that he was sorry that my job had been eliminated, and I hurried to leave so that I would not say or do something that I would regret. It took less than thirty minutes. I stopped at the office to clean out my desk, and as I drove home, I rehearsed how I would explain this to Mary. She would have no warning. Sometimes the changes in life are gradual. This one was like a lightening bolt.

So, what do you do when you are forty-five years old, have two kids in college, and all of a sudden have a career of twenty-two years end? I didn't know the answer to the question. I had always had good employee benefits, not really giving the issue of insurance coverage a second thought. As I began to collect my thoughts, and look at paperwork provided to me, I felt shaken, vulnerable. My doctor had said I had a terminal illness and the coverage I had enjoyed would only last a little while. I knew I was uninsurable. And technology was changing just as fast as the lightening bolt. What would I do?

Now that I look back on that time, which seemed so awful, God has given me some reflection and insight. I had to get out of the stress and pressure of traveling every week. I could not see the changes in my heart at the time, but I now realize that all of the "push" was slowly but surely weakening my heart and hastening the inevitable day when I would be in heart failure. That I was forced out of that pressure-packed grind was God's grace, bringing an abrupt change in lifestyle that I would never have initiated myself.

Being out of work was not stress-free however. Fortunately, God clearly had already set in motion some positive help before we knew it was needed. Rachel was the student at Wake Forest chosen for a grant that enabled her to leave in August, which was within a few weeks, to spend her junior year in Kiev, Ukraine in the old Soviet Union. The grant covered all her costs, including airfare. The very week that she was to leave, the political coup happened in Moscow. She was adamant that she was going. She was a dreamer as a twenty-year-old, just like her dad had been. This was before the days of easy internet use or cell phones. We had been told that after we put her on the plane, we would not hear from her for six weeks. There were very few Americans in Kiev. Fortunately she was good at the Russian language, so she made it just fine. We managed to make it somehow. The way we heard from her was a five-minute phone call that she had to schedule at the post office in Kiev. The schedule was not reliable, and she did not know for sure when she went if a call would go through. When it finally worked, it was such a relief to hear her voice! By the time she flew back to the states for Christmas, we would have heard from her only three times.

There had been big changes in David's life earlier in this same tumultuous year of 1991. We had been proud that he had graduated as a National Merit Scholar, which precipitated the full scholarship to Texas A&M. David loved the Aggie "bull," all the bonfire activities, and friends. But he was not headed in the right career direction. This fact emerged painfully, as he made both A's and F's. If the class had appeal to him, he was passionate; but the classes with hundreds of students where there was no actual relationship with a "prof" turned him off. He just skipped the class. We only discovered later that he was a hard core "mentor" learner who relished the challenge of a mentor who was as much a friend as a professor. While he had great technical and science skills, he was, at heart, an artist, and, unknown to us, secretly desired to be a commercial photographer.

The roller-coaster effort ended David's stay at Texas A&M. He spent a semester as a volunteer at the Gano Street Mission Center in inner-city Houston, founded by Mildred McWhorter. During these months, he saw the worst side of life, poverty, and trouble. It proved to be an important time in his life as he came to grips with how God was working in him.

Mary and I had given him his first camera that we bought used at a camera shop when he was eleven years old. He already had a great deal of photography knowledge and ability. He asked us to affirm who he was and what he wanted to do. He had friends who told him that if he went the "commercial photography" direction, he would be "wasting his life." Mary and I began to understand, though it was difficult for us. I was sure that if he really wanted to, he could be a great scientist or technician. It took time for me to understand that he was an artist. He inherited that from his mother, I believe.

David explained that there were three schools in the country that offered a Bachelor of Fine Arts degree in commercial photography. The one in the eastern part of the country was Rochester Institute of Technology, where Eastman Kodak is located. The one on the west coast was Brooks Institute in Santa

Barbara, California. The third one was the Center for Creative Studies in Detroit, Michigan. Although it was very expensive, CCS was the least expensive of the three and in January of 1991, Mary and I drove Dave to DFW and put him on a plane to Detroit to begin his time at CCS. He had never been there and did not know anyone there.

Thus, by September of 1991, Rachel was in Kiev and David was in Detroit. We were in Denton and I had no job! What was happening to my dreams, our dreams?

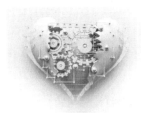

LIVING ON THE EDGE

The day I went to Texas Employment Commission to file for unemployment is a memorable one. I had always been motivated and successful. Here I was in a room full of people who did not have jobs. As I looked around, all I could hear in my thoughts was *"Failure!"* In my inner thoughts, I asked God how I had gotten to such a place. Many past moments came into my thought-life as I sat there waiting.

I had a heritage of faith and had gone to church all my life. But I had not always had a devotional life, that sense of inner peace and intimacy with a God who loved me and cared for me. Sometimes I went through the motions spiritually. When David and Rachel were still very young, one day I came home for lunch and noticed on our refrigerator that Mary had written out a scripture verse and had it out where she could see it. She bought a Living Bible and read it faithfully. She was involved with a group of young mothers who shared and studied and prayed. She was developing a devotional life, believing that prayer was real and powerful. That wasn't really happening with me. I had an academic faith. I had studied at the seminary and knew something about the Bible. But I did not have the devotional passion that was emerging in Mary. I wanted it. I wanted to believe that

God was near and that I really knew Him, that I had a relationship on the inside, and that when I prayed, it really mattered.

I saw that in Mary in so many ways. When the children were small, I had a "moonlight" business of doing landscape work on evenings and Saturdays. Sometimes in Texas it is so hot! On the hottest Saturday in July, I had an all-day job to take care of a large lawn and many flower beds for a business. There was no shade and perspiration was pouring off of me. I looked up to see Mary and David and Rachel driving up to bring me something cool to drink. It was so refreshing. Mary saw how hot I was and how I was laboring in the heat, and before she left she said, "I am going to pray that God will put a little cloud over you to give you some *shade*." Soon she was gone and I was working away. In a few minutes, I realized that I was cooler than I had been. Then I looked up and saw that there was a little cloud that had me in the shade! It was amazing. I worked the rest of the afternoon in the shade of that small cloud.

So, if she had simple, devotional faith that seemed to make a difference, why shouldn't I? I too began to pick up the Bible and read it devotionally. As I did so, I wondered if I might also have a more meaningful prayer life, something beyond just reciting familiar phrases over and over. I realized that prayer needed to be more of a lifestyle that went on inside me through the day, rather that something I just said at certain times like before meals. So I began to write a verse of scripture on my desk calendar at work each day. My days were busy and I had lots of important projects with deadlines, but somehow it was nice just to pause momentarily and reflect on the verse. Some days I would try to memorize the verse. While it was good for me, it never occurred to me that God might be doing *something beyond me* in the process.

So much of my spiritual life seemed all about me. In those days, to implement some of the new computer applications on the mainframe, we had to come in deep in the night or on weekends to have the dedicated system time to do our implementation. It was on such an occasion that I happened to be sitting at my desk in the wee hours one morning. I was startled by a man who came around the corner to face my desk. I could see that he was startled to see me there. I had never seen him before. He said he was the night janitor. He asked if that was my desk, and I told him that it was. Then he made an amazing statement to me. "I don't have much education, and I have trouble finding things in the Bible. But for several months I have been stopping at your desk each night and God always seems to have a good word for me, written out on your calendar." That moment was foundational in my life. I came to understand that God is always at work around me, whether I can see it or not. I just needed to be faithful to do the right thing and trust God to be at work, even if I couldn't see it.

Prayer became a routine part of my life at home, and I constantly asked God what he wanted me to do with my life, and how I should lead my family. One morning I woke up and realized that I had just had a very vivid and meaningful dream that seemed to be responding to my prayers. This was not a normal occurrence for me. I pondered the dream. In it, the current sheriff of Denton County, Wylie Barnes, was on a railroad platform beckoning to me to come and help him. The solid conviction that came was that God wanted me to go to the Denton County jail and share out of my new growing devotional relationship with the Lord. But quickly I remembered a hot Sunday afternoon many years before when I had left the same Denton County jail in shame, swearing in my heart that I would never go back there. It was another crisis of belief.

However, there was such a compelling sense about the dream that I knew I had to do something. The next Saturday morning

I went to the jail and met the jailer on duty. I told him that I thought God wanted me to share with the men at the jail. He really didn't say much to me. He just motioned for me to follow him into the elevator and before long I was standing in front of the "drunk tank," which was overflowing from lots of Friday-night partying. The men looked at me and I realized that I did have something to say out of the new devotional relationship with Jesus Christ that was growing in me. What commenced that day led to more than thirty-two years of jail ministry!

So that job and those early foundational days in my devotional life were long gone and just became good memories in my thought-life. I was back in the unemployment office, faced with the defeated and failing sense of being unemployed. But I was not dealing with that alone. Since those times all those years before, I had this inner thought-life relationship with God Himself! While there was discouragement and fear, there was still a strong internal peace and assurance that God was at work. I just could not see Him or see how He was working. And that is the essence of faith: believing and knowing, without being able to see.

Soon I was drawing unemployment checks and sending out resumes. Nothing opened up. We knew that there was a parent's weekend at CCS in October in Detroit, so we decided that since we had the time, we would drive to Detroit from Texas for that weekend. Along the way we had the first occasion to visit Louisville, Kentucky, since our early married days when we had left twenty-two years before to move back to Texas. We went on to visit my sister Jo and her husband Jack who were involved in ministry in Ohio. We went on to Niagara Falls, and drove back along the Canadian side to Detroit. It was so good to see David in this new situation. The photography program was obviously good, and he was so pleased to show us around and introduce us to friends he had met. There were only a few hundred students and he seemed to have strong relationships with all his mentors. For a while, we forgot about the jobless state that I was in and just enjoyed the trip.

When we returned to Texas, reality descended on me, and I fought worry and anxiety about our future. I never ever thought about my natural heart and the possibility that it might get progressively worse.

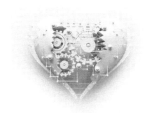

STARTING OVER

Mary and I began to consider the possibility that this would be the time of a really substantial change in our whole life, not just another position in another company, but a career change. We were familiar with the crossroads moments. They always seemed to come. By this time, we had done the "Experiencing God" study by Henry Blackaby. In this study, he describes such a crossroads moment as a "Crisis of Belief."

Because of my aptitudes and the conversations with some friends, I began to consider the possibility of becoming a financial advisor. The statistics were not particularly optimistic. Only one in ten people who started down this path were still in the business a year later. Such a direction did not offer immediate benefits as a regular corporate job did. I was uninsurable and soon would be without any insurance coverage (this was before the best of the days of COBRA). But I seemed to have the aptitude and was more and more drawn in that direction.

There were some hurdles. It was a business that took a long time to build an income stream, and we had a lot of financial responsibilities that seemed to demand immediate regular income. Most of the opportunities in that field seemed to be in Dallas, and we had deep roots in Denton and wanted to stay put where we were. It was a business that would require a lot of up-front preparation and lots of study to secure and maintain licenses and affiliations.

Such was the situation late one afternoon when I had an interview with a man in Dallas named John Lovick, a Firm Director with John Hancock with many years in the business. We spent more than two hours just talking. He asked what I really wanted to do in life, and I responded, "just to please God." My unusual response seemed to open our conversation to a deeper level. John had no problem with me building a practice in Denton. He had every assurance that I would do well in the long run and somehow support my family from the beginning. That long session let to the eighteen-year career that I am now in!

But it wasn't easy. I began to work seventy- and eighty-hour weeks, getting all the training and licenses, and setting the stage to begin my practice. I discovered why only one in ten survives the first year. On one occasion, I pulled an "all-nighter" just to do a task that I was told had to be done. Yet, more than three months later when I finally received my first income, I was shocked to see that my first net pay was $75. My unemployment was running out, I had no insurance coverage, and I was working as hard as I knew how to work. It truly was a crisis of belief. Had I somehow made a mistake and gone down the wrong path? Mary and I constantly prayed and asked God for His direction and for a way to make it through this.

We scraped by financially week by week. We held our breath about health issues, knowing that it would take six months in order for my contract to grant me any kind of group medical insurance. In spite of the struggle, I found myself very much fulfilled in what I was doing and sure that I was having a positive impact in other people's lives.

Then an option came out of the blue that we never expected. I got a call from Pete Harvey, Vice President of Sales for Moore

Business Forms. He wanted to talk to me about a new position that he felt I was uniquely qualified for. I had a long meeting with him. He expressed regret at how I had been treated the year before and indicated that those who knew me had kept me in mind when new opportunities opened up. He wanted me to fly to the Research Division of Moore at Grand Island, New York, and have a look at some new technology that would be my area of responsibility. I made the trip within the next two days, and then came home to spend the day with Mary considering what we should do before my scheduled meeting back with Pete the next day.

On the surface, this new option seemed to be a God thing. All my benefits and tenure would be immediately restored, and I would make more in income than I had been making when I left. It seemed to mean that in one week I would be delivered from uncertainty and scraping by to the full and immediate restoration of all my benefits and the return of a long and good career, with a good income. What was there to even think about? Yet, as we talked that afternoon, Mary shared that she had seen much fulfillment in me from doing the work I was now doing. It was nice to have me at home and not always traveling somewhere. She remembered the grind and all the travel of the past.

The very one of us who would typically feel the need for security, Mary, finally said that she felt that I should continue with what I was now doing, trusting God to answer all the uncertainties, since that seemed to be what He wanted. I would never have had the courage to turn down such an option without her strong encouragement. The next afternoon, I met with Pete Harvey and expressed my appreciation for the opportunity, and then declined the offer. He could not believe that I did not accept the offer. However, it brought to Mary and I, as a couple, the strong sense that now we were doing what we were doing by choice, and not because we were forced to. In spite of the uncertainty, there came a new freedom in our thought-life as we trusted what we believed but could not see.

I always enjoyed listening to Paul Harvey's *The Rest of the Story* on the radio. The rest of this story is fascinating. When I declined the offer from Pete Harvey, he asked if I knew of anyone who had the unique set of skills this new position required. At the time, our friends Tom and Betty Hickey were in a crossroads moment in their life. Tom had spent twenty-five years with IBM and was being asked to relocate to Tulsa, Oklahoma. Tom would be ideal for the job, I thought. Mary and I called Tom and Betty and we met at the Dairy Queen to have a Blizzard. I asked Tom if he might want to consider the opportunity with Moore and avoid the move. Quickly Tom interviewed with Pete Harvey and was soon working in this new position. Three years later, Tom called me one afternoon, distressed and disconsolate. That afternoon a new manager who had been brought into the organization had called Tom in and fired him. He collected his company car keys and told him to clean out his desk. There would be a taxi to drive him home within the hour! How fleeting "security" is in this life. Truly God had led Mary and me in rejecting the offer. God could see beyond the relief of the moment the position seemed to offer and to the purpose of the future. We are still living the "rest of the story."

Some stories have a "they lived happily ever after" kind of ending. Ours does, I believe. Looking back through the years to that time, we see that we made the right decision, and we have had much joy and lots of good times. But it we did not immediately result in a smooth path. We have had many challenges. Our business did come along, but we did not quickly have financial security. In fact, I found myself, nine months later, realizing that I would have to call David in Detroit and tell him that I did not see how we would be able to pay his tuition in the fall. I dreaded doing that, knowing that he was on the right path in his life and was working hard, himself. He had gotten some photography jobs to help financially, and by this point he was a Resident Assistant in the one CCS dorm.

David had always had such simple and strong faith, like his mother. His temperament was like Mary's–relaxed and easy. I called him and explained the situation. He simply said, "Dad, we prayed before I came to CCS that it was the right thing. And it is. God will make a way." After we finished the conversation, I found myself thinking that David really just didn't "get it," the seriousness of our situation. I certainly did not see any way to cover a very large tuition payment in a few months! In the realm of what I could see, it would be an inexplicable miracle for him to be in school at CCS the next fall.

A few weeks later David called me and I could sense that something encouraging was going on. He told me how that CCS had bought a new film processor from Kodak, and he had asked the head of the photography department, Dr. Vigiletti, who was going to install the processor. Dr. Vigiletti told him that Kodak would be contracted to do the installation. He found out that CCS would be paying a thousand dollars for the installation. Dave then had approached Dr. Vigiletti and told him that he would do the installation for $500. CCS had contracted with him and he had done the installation. I asked David how he knew how to do the installation, and he said, "Dad, it came with a manual!" Then he explained that the manager of the photography lab had left CCS, and Dr. Vigiletti had discussed with David the possibility of taking over the position. He thought the $8.35 per hour was good pay, and he would be allowed to work his classes in. I could quickly compute that the hourly income would help David pay for gas and expenses, but it could not even make a dent in the $11,000 per semester tuition. Then he dropped the critical information. "Dad, they consider this a faculty position, and for faculty, they waive tuition!" I was overwhelmed at David's simple faith, and at God's confirmation and provision for David's direction in life. It was a faith-building time. We did not have a clue, however, at the amount of faith that would eventually be required in David's life.

We were able to visit David in Detroit several times. His primary mentor was a faculty member named Fred Crudder. Fred and his wife, Sally, had one of the old palatial homes in a historic area of Detroit not far from CCS. Some of these homes dated back to the late 1800s and were owned by the elite wealthy families of Detroit. They had "carriage houses," where the carriages were stored, and they had side entrances where the owners could get directly into or out of their carriages. Fred's house was such a place. He constantly had renovation projects going, and David had all the skills and was at Fred's side throughout the renovation process. Dave lived in the carriage house behind Fred's house, and Mary and I came to see him for the first time there. We had to climb stairs to a landing and then climb another set of stairs the rest of the way to David's apartment.

When we reached the landing, Mary looked out the window by the landing and asked David why there was a small round hole in the window. David told us that there was a drug house across the alley. This neighborhood was in transition, and there was a lot of violence and unlawful activity taking place there. There was sometimes gunfire, and the landing window had taken a direct hit. So much for Mom's reassurance about her son's safety! He later called me back in Texas and reported that his car had been stolen but had been found. When it was retrieved, it was stripped and missing from inside was some photography equipment that belonged to CCS. An enterprising and street-wise policeman helped him retrieve the equipment within the hour from a pawn shop. Thankfully, it got returned to CCS, but his prized Panasonic car stereo system was never located. So went life with a "mentor learner."

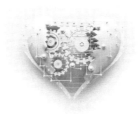

WORLD TRAVELER

Rachel is like me in many ways, just as David had many of his mother's traits. She seemed an aggressive dreamer, always pushing the envelope.

She finished her degree at Wake Forest, and immediately had a job with Occidental Petroleum in Siberia. It seemed like a fast-forward movie, almost before we knew what was happening; she was somewhere called Nizhnevartovsk, in remote Siberia, where there was only wasteland and oil drilling. Soon there were stories of helicopter rides into the arctic circle in bitter cold. Actually, when I think about it, that sounds like a bad dream and not a fulfilling one!

The stark and lonely life was too much for her, so her next stop was Moscow, where she rented a flat and worked for first one and then another telecommunications company, trying to break into the emerging Russian business life. She had a driver, and later we found out that the way she helped get the businesses started in Moscow was by purchasing computers and office equipment on the black market, often carrying large sums of cash on her in order to get around the endless delays that came with working through the regular "system." On Sundays, she was very involved in a church that included both Russians and Americans, so the service had to be translated. She has an unusual language skill and native fluency in Russian, so she was the one to translate into English when a Russian pastor preached. In 1995, we were blessed to be able to spend three weeks in Russia, staying with Rachel in her flat. We toured around in the day while she was at work.

It was such a challenging place to live and get around. There were none of the ordinary conveniences, never any ice on the hot summer days; life was just so brutal. (Actually, Rachel reminded us that there was lots of ice on the streets in the winter!) We learned to take the metro and I memorized the Russian letters for the metro stops. The people on the metro were so sad and unhappy looking, always looking down or away and never making eye contract. We took a tour of the Kremlin, saw Red Square, saw the Russian ballet, and went to church and listened to a blind Russian pastor preach as Rachel stood beside him and translated into English.

On the weekend Rachel was available to go with us on an overnight train ride to St. Petersburg. The railway stations are hard to describe. There was only one "eastern" toilet, which made us determined to "just hold it." There are so many alcoholics that the halls of the stations were full of people passed out, and we had to gingerly tiptoe over and around them.

I am sure Rachel didn't want to alarm me, so she did not tell me ahead of time about our "first class" accommodations on the train. When we boarded, we walked down a long hall and she said to me, "This compartment is for Mom and me. Yours is the next one. There will likely be another man in the compartment with you." Only at that moment did I realize that I was about to be sharing a very small compartment with a cot that folded down on each side, and that some Russian stranger might sleep just across from me, a couple of feet away! Sure enough, in a few minutes a Russian man came into the compartment. He had on a tee-shirt that said "Georgia Baptist Hospital" on it.

He was delighted to have an American sharing his compartment, giving him an opportunity to practice his English. It turned out that he and his wife were both doctors, and that he was the medical director of the hospital in St. Petersburg, returning after a meeting in Moscow. He told me about his daughter, who was in medical school in America, and he softly confided about the sad state of medicine in Russia. He pulled out his bottle of vodka and invited me to join him. When I declined, he put it up and we spent most of our trip talking. I learned that many Russian professional families only have one child and that most Russian women have had multiple abortions. I got a fascinating look at Russian life, outside the normal tourist stops.

Rachel flew to Detroit to meet us for David's graduation from CCS in 1994. He had already been working as the photo lab manager for Midcoast Studios. Midcoast was a major photography studio that specialized in doing photography projects for the big automobile makers such as GM and Chrysler and also for Harley Davidson motorcycles. We were worried that David seemed in a too-serious relationship with a Detroit girl. With the prospects of such good work at what he loved to do in Detroit, and with Rachel working in Russia, Mary and I began to come to grips with the possibility that both our kids might, for the rest of their lives, live very far away from us.

The next year, David found a cheap flight from Chicago to Moscow on Aeroflot and spent a week in Moscow with Rachel. There were new war stories to be told in the family about how David got lost in Moscow on his way to meet Rachel at the circus (he didn't speak Russian). She was amazed that somehow he found his way. It still is not clear to any of us how that happened.

Some of the very best of David's photography are some black and white shots that he made in Moscow. They are great memories.

Some of the family wanderlust seemed to settle on David, and he began to talk about taking a backpacking photography tour of Alaska. He would continue to work in Detroit for another year, but in August, 1996, David came to Denton and started collecting the supplies that he would need for a forty day backpacking trek, *alone*, to Alaska. I enjoyed studying the maps and reading with him about the various places that he wanted to go. The basic plan was to maintain a locker in a youth hostel in Anchorage. Then each week he would catch a flight on a float-plane to one of the isolated areas he wanted to photograph. He would backpack through that area for a week and then catch the float-plane back to Anchorage, where he would restock his backpack from the stash in the locker and then head to the next area.

He made stops near Denali, getting a clear picture unobstructed by clouds, which was very unusual. He would get to the "Valley of 10,000 Smokes." However, he would be discouraged by a sprained ankle, loneliness, and a lost camera and film. He would later tell his Granny Earp about a dark, lonely night when he rediscovered his faith that he had put on hold in his life. He was glad to get home and then return to Detroit to work. He did not develop a passion to go back to Alaska.

However, David's Alaska photography graces the walls of the patient waiting area of the Bone Marrow Transplant offices in Collins Hospital at Baylor Medical Center in Dallas, where David was a patient for so long. Every time I return to that area, though there are sad and painful memories, they make the place seem all "David." I can sit in the room and see the photos and immediately feel Dave and all the stories rush back. I wish I had been with him in Alaska.

The same year that David went to Alaska, Rachel decided that she would leave Moscow, but would make one last grand trip to all the places that she had heard about, but never been. She had a friend whom she had met through the U.S. Embassy activities in Moscow, a young woman about Rachel's age, who was also from Texas and was just as adventurous as Rachel. They decided to backpack throughout Asia, carrying with them only the items in their backpacks. They flew from Moscow to Beijing and toured China, walking on the Great Wall. They would go to Hong Kong, Singapore, Indonesia, and Bangkok before stopping in India to see the Taj Mahal. Then they flew through Dubai on their way to Cairo, where they went to the Great Pyramids and the Valley of the Kings. While in Cairo, there was political turmoil due to the assassination of the Israeli prime minister.

They had plans to take the bus across the Sinai to Jerusalem, but Rachel's friend decided she had had enough and took a flight back to Moscow. So alone and with only her backpack for a companion, Rachel determined to take the bus to Jerusalem. She stayed at a retreat center and had a wonderful, contemplative week walking to the sites that had such spiritual significance.

While there, she took some striking black and white pictures. She kept a journal, and one of my most prized possessions is a book that she made and gave to me as a gift with the pictures matched up with her meditations at the location of each picture. When she got to Tel Aviv to take her flight back to Moscow, she was detained by security for four hours. Israeli officials are very careful about security, and her passport was so full of stops that they thought surely there must have been something suspicious about all her travels! By the end of the year, she would leave Moscow to head home to rest up for a few weeks before heading to a new life in Washington D.C.

Rachel went on to live a very significant six years in Washington D.C. She worked as a civilian analyst for the Department of Defense. She earned a national level award in 1999. She served two tours in Bosnia, Serbia, and Croatia during this time of her life. As a fluent native Russian-speaker, Rachel had a leg-up in learning the Serbo-Croatian language. When she arrived for her first tour in Tuzla, she had already gone through intense training at Fort Huachuca in the Arizona desert, and had learned to shoot at a DOD facility in Virginia. While at Tuzla, she debriefed the townspeople in small villages who told her stories of the carnage and murder in the villages by the opposing ethnic cultures.

Rachel and her team were housed in a non-descript neighborhood near the Tuzla military base. Her closest call came one night when she was alone and realized there was an intruder in the dark of the apartment. Only by the grace of God was she able to escape out the window and climb a very tall fence.

After a few months of rest and relaxation back in Washington, D.C., Rachel returned for her second tour, being based in Sarajevo the whole time. The first night she was on base, she was in the shower, and there came a knock on the door. It was after 10 p.m. and she was exhausted from the long trip from the states. When she opened the door, the colonel who was the chief of staff for the commanding general of the stabilization force in Bosnia (SFOR) was there. He rushed her to get ready to go on an urgent and unexpected mission.

The SFOR commander routinely had high-level meetings with heads of state all over Bosnia. Rachel was always a part of his entourage, a striking young blonde dressed in military fatigues at the general's side. When this tour was over, the commander sent to Mary and me a most prized possession: a large, official engraved plaque with a black and white photo of Rachel with her helmet and headphones onboard the helicopter. The caption on the plaque expressed the General's gratitude to us for allowing Rachel to serve in such a strategic and unusual way.

Upon her return to Washington D.C., Rachel fulfilled a long-term educational dream, earning her Master's degree in International Intelligence from Georgetown University. Mary and I were blessed to be in attendance at Georgetown the day she received her graduate degree.

We enjoyed visiting Rachel. She had an apartment in Arlington, Virginia, not far from the Pentagon. She and Mary enjoyed shopping at the Pentagon mall, and that gave me the chance to visit, or revisit, one of the civil war battle sites in the area. I have been able to spend time at Gettysburg on seven different occasions. Rachel was always involved in church, and we always were encouraged by going to church with her. We would often eat breakfast at the Metro diner not far from Fort Myer, and we never missed driving down to Mt. Vernon for lunch. What a blessing!

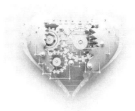

TEXAS, OUR TEXAS!

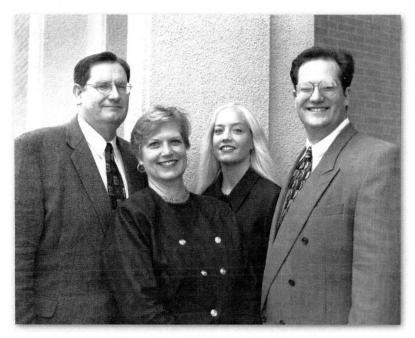

James, Mary, Rachel, and David –
healthy and doing well in front of our church

After David had gone through his graduation ceremony at CCS in 1994, he reluctantly told us that the diploma received was not real. He had an "incomplete" in an English class, due to a paper that had not been done. He rationalized that it really didn't matter, as he had a great job and no one in the commercial photography world really cared about an English paper. He was moving quickly to the next exciting phase of his life and had no intention of spending time on an English paper! He was correct that no one at Midcoast Studios seemed concerned in the least about this issue. But to Mary and me, the actual degree mattered.

So Mary began a ceaseless effort to motivate David to take care of the issue so that he would have a real diploma and the long-hoped-for degree. Life was busy and good for David, and one semester passed, and then a year, without any action toward dealing with the matter. Mary was relentless, using every chance she had to talk to David as an opportunity to go back to the issue. It didn't help that he lived 1,300 miles from us and was constantly on the go with lots of projects going on.

He loved the camaraderie and close fellowship of doing a "shoot" as the crew would go to Milwaukee for a shoot for Harley Davidson, or go to Arizona each spring to do the Chevrolet Suburban shoot. They would start in Arizona, shooting through California and Oregon, before ending up in the state of Washington. We were pleased and surprised finally to hear that he had paid the tuition to retake the course the spring semester of 1996. The required paper was done at the last minute, on the road, as he faxed the paper in to CCS from Arizona. He finally got a real diploma, but fussed when he received it, since it showed the degree being conferred in 1996, rather than his original graduation day in 1994.

He began to talk about moving back to Texas to work more on his own as an individual photographer. He now had the degree, he had done his dream backpacking trip, and he had done lots of projects with Midcoast. He seemed ready to move on to the next phase of his life. Starting over in a total new area (where he was unknown professionally) promised to be tough, and we encouraged him to do it sooner than later. We had heard about the "revolving door," with adult children coming back home. It was now our turn to install a "revolving door." We actually thought it would be great to have him around, and invited him to move back to Texas and into his old bedroom. So, in September, 1997, he pulled into our driveway with his Suburban loaded to the ceiling with all of his stuff. It was wonderful to have him back.

Now that the diploma issue had been settled, Mary began to work on David about the church issue. We knew that his faith had been renewed in the darkness and loneliness of Alaska, but he never really got into a church in the six years he lived in Detroit. While growing up in a family of faith is good, every person has to eventually own their own faith. If it is real, it cannot be inherited. Mary did her best to convince David that as he was "starting over," he should now go back to church.

Just down the hall from where our Bible class met, there was a "Professional Singles" class. The director of this group was a very nice math teacher named DLynn Tatum. Mary encouraged David to try this group out. He reluctantly gave in to his mother's wishes, and on the first Sunday back in Texas, he visited this group. Not much was said about it. The next Friday evening when I arrived back at our home, David was walking out the door, splashing on cologne. I asked him where he was going, and he replied, "to Bible study!"

He became a regular in the group and made good friends. Within just six weeks, it occurred to us that DLynn might be more than just a new friend. She had grown up in Louisiana and had gotten her degree from Louisiana Tech. She had a family connection with Barbara Fischer, a school principal in Denton who needed a math teacher. Just a year before, DLynn had become a Texan. She was a strong believer, and soon was leading her group at our church. David's interest in Bible study and "Christian fellowship" ebbed, and by Thanksgiving, we could see where their relationship was headed. David quickly left our Christmas visiting to make a trip to Louisiana to see DLynn and meet her family.

In January, he carefully orchestrated a unique proposal. He lined signs along the route that DLynn took home from school, with the last sign spelling out his proposal of marriage and with him standing beside the sign with a dozen roses in his hand. The spring of 1998 was an exciting time for us, as we got to know DLynn more and were involved in the planning of a wedding.

Except, it would not be just any wedding. It was one to remember, adding a whole new library of family lore and funny stories. They chose as their wedding day Saturday, June 13, 1998. David and DLynn would make their wedding true to their unique personalities, bypassing the traditional church wedding. They decided to get married before a small group of family and friends under the shade of a very large tree in the Denton City Park. The beautiful area is surrounded by shrubbery and flowers and has a small bridge in the background. They signed the paperwork and made the deposit that would allow them to use the park. David was known for the uniqueness and complexity of his projects, so two "Dave" projects ensued.

First, he decided that the perfect cover for the ceremony would be a large, lattice-like canopy covered in greenery and anchored to two large wooden pedestals. Joined by some of his friends from Detroit who came for the wedding, the driveway behind our house became a "canopy construction zone." The canopy would have to be assembled at the park, and then immediately after the wedding in the park, moved quickly to the fellowship hall of our church where the reception would be held. The wild card in this was that the day of the wedding was the hottest June day in recent memory. The temperature topped out at 110 degrees that day! So Dave's Uncle Wes and Uncle Bill were exhausted in the heat as they rushed to help move the canopy to the church.

The other project was unknown to Mary and me at the time. It unfolded the night before the wedding. Dave decided that the setting in the park was perfect for the wedding, with one exception. Somehow the color of the bridge in the park did not match the color theme of the wedding photography, so during that night he and DLynn repainted the bridge so that the color would be right for the pictures!

The wedding was beautiful in spite of the heat. We were blessed with a large group of family and friends at the reception. The major challenge for Dave and DLynn was that their rented limo's air conditioner was not working! Things got back to normal while they were gone. Their deposit was sacrificed to the city for the bridge painting, and the canopy was returned to the yard at our house for us to figure out what to do with.

They returned from their honeymoon to their little home that they had just bought in Denton. Sometimes when telling stories, we end with "and they lived happily ever after." Recently my eight-year-old granddaughter, Tatum, and I were driving and we had on one of our favorite children's song CDs with a song that says, "I'm happy all the time." Tatum said to me, "Grampsie, that song is wrong, we are not always happy." I acknowledged her wisdom beyond her years. She understood that happiness is based on circumstances, and circumstances are sometimes bad. So we discussed the difference between *joy*, an attitude on the inside that, by God's grace, sees us through all bad circumstances and *happiness* on the outside, which seems dependent on circumstances. Now that we know what the journey that Dave and DLynn would travel was like, it would be truthful to say "they lived *joyfully* ever after." Their pre-wedding bridge painting project was just a taste of things to come. They loved spending time together at Lowe's, getting the materials that they needed to do a series of projects on their house. Soon projects were not just "Dave projects," they were "Dave and DLynn projects." They had endless, often perfectionist, ideas about how things should be. And they had such an unusual term of endearment for each other, "Homey." It was fun to watch!

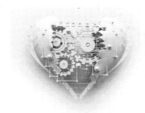

A GOOD YEAR

The year 2000 was a good year for Mary and me. We were able to make several trips and have impact in a variety of ways through our church and missions projects and through our Bible class. In January, I made a mission trip to Haiti. Although I have been there a number of times, traveling there seemed to be increasingly dangerous.

Our first trip to Haiti had occurred several years before, when our new pastor, Dr. Jeff Williams, had stated in his plans for his first year as our pastor the "ten things he wanted to do that year." One of the ten things he indicated he wanted to do was to take a mission trip. The Monday morning after that Sunday, I knocked on his office door and asked if he would consider making a mission trip to Haiti. After a few weeks he called me back and said he would. Two months later Dr. Jeff, Roger Frederick, John Duncan, and I found ourselves for the very first time in the challenging and dangerous country of Haiti. We were hosted by our friends Dr. Jacob and Claudette Bernard, who are natives of Haiti, but who, with their five children, spent many years in Boston, in Florida, and then in Texas getting a variety of degrees in preparation for a lifetime of ministry in Haiti. The Bernards had moved to Haiti in 1991, after laboring for years to try to raise support.

Finally, Jacob decided that he would take his family and move without the needed support. Jacob's brother especially opposed their return to Haiti, due to the severe life there. In an effort to abort this family move to Haiti, when they were at the Miami airport waiting to board the outbound flight to Port-au-Prince, Jacob's brother called the Miami police and begged them to arrest Jacob, as it seemed the only way to stop them!

Years of extreme hardship and testing ensued for them. I felt called to support them, but the meager amounts raised barely sustained them at a poverty level. My hopes were buoyed now that my new pastor had finally led a small group of us to go there.

Through Dr. Jeff's leadership, our future trips involved groups of students and a few sponsors working on construction and ministry projects. This initial trip was small in scope but strategic in planning for the future. Dr. Jeff had preached on Sunday morning to a packed Bolosse Baptist Church in Port-au-Prince, with more than 2,500 people in attendance.

Our next trip in 1999 was Brad Cockrell's first. He was the student minister at our church, and would eventually be instrumental in several of the student groups going. Mary and I and all the rest were adult laypeople. We traveled on rough roads to the rural interior of Haiti, which was very different from the squalor and steaming masses of people in Port-au-Prince. The poverty was overwhelming and the illnesses from malnutrition and polluted drinking water contributed to a fragile and often short life for the Haitians.

We finally arrived in the most remote area where the Albert Switzer Hospital was. As we walked through the operating room, we were surprised to see chickens and goats leisurely walking among the operating tables and hospital beds. There were clothes lines with dozens of surgical gloves that were hanging to dry so they could be reused! One outcome of the trip was a strong conviction that we could do more to bring medical supplies and medications in when we came.

By the time we were returning to Port-au-Prince, it was in the heat of the afternoon and was absolutely hot even though it was January. Our driver pulled our van into the open market in a small village to give the van a rest. The villagers immediately surrounded our van, begging for food. We had the windows rolled up in the van and were shouting to one another that it was not wise to lower the windows, as the people seemed as if they would climb in the van with us. We always traveled with bottled water and snacks such as peanuts or crackers, knowing there would not be a safe place to eat on our day-long journeys. A young mother, perhaps fourteen years old, stood outside the window where Brad was sitting. She held a crying baby who displayed the physical evidence of malnutrition: tinged red hair and a protruding stomach. As she begged at the window, Brad exclaimed that he could not emotionally handle our "hoarding" our snacks in the midst of such need. So we devised a strategy: we would all get snacks into our hands and roll the windows down briefly just as the driver was driving away. We prayed for God to help us and then quickly handed our leftovers out the windows as the driver sped away. We looked back to see the young mother and the baby with crackers in each hand hungrily taking a bite from first one hand and then the other. It would be a moment in time that would forever impact my life and my outlook, somehow seeing the desperate needs of fellow human beings, *real people,* through the loving eyes and hands of God himself.

Back in the states, Mary and I traveled to business conferences in California and Boston, and we took our longest vacation ever, a trip to the Pacific Northwest that included stops in Seattle. We went to Vancouver, Whistler, Victoria, Mount

Rainer, Seaside, Fort Clatsop, and Astoria in Oregon and some of the lighthouses along the Pacific coast.

In July, Rachel had a very sad event in her life. Her dear friend Andrea, a young lawyer who lived not far from Rachel, died of lung cancer. Andrea had never smoked, but was afflicted with the disease, nonetheless. Rachel had been there with Andrea as she had many kinds of treatment and finally a lung transplant. In the end, she died as a young woman in her early thirties. Rachel flew to Michigan to be with her family and to speak at her memorial service. It seems to me that this sad loss put a fog over Rachel's enthusiasm to live and work in Washington D.C.

Perhaps as a form of therapy, Rachel informed us that she had decided to train to run in the twenty-fifth running of the Marine Corps marathon in Washington D.C. In October we flew to Washington D.C. for the marathon. What an amazing day it was as we mapped out a plan to ride the metro to several key locations to observe Rachel as she came by, and then to see her at the finish near the Iwo Jima memorial. The weather was great and there were more than 25,000 participants. It was a sight to see the flood of runners running along the Potomac with the Pentagon and Arlington National Cemetery in the background. There were a couple of challenges: we miscalculated and missed Rachel at a couple of places, and at about mile fourteen, she had a fall, but got up quickly and continued. We were so proud to see her coming up the final hill to the finish line. She finished about 12,000[th] out of the more than 25,000, with a time of a little over five hours. How exciting!

Increasingly, we understood that though she had traveled many places and done many things, Rachel was lonely and wanted to be married and have a family. The loss of her friend Andrea seemed to cause a different kind of perspective about what God wanted to do in her life. These emerging desires of her heart had us in constant prayer that God might grant them.

We enjoyed our family Thanksgiving celebration in Floydada, Texas. My father had died in 1984, at the age of seventy-four and my mother had eventually moved to Floydada to live near my sister, Molly. Our family Thanksgiving times were celebrations as we ate and played "42" and shared openly and joyfully and watched Dallas Cowboys football. All the cousins wanted Granny as their "42" partner. She was such a pleasant, smiling person who so enjoyed those times. This would be her last with us. She was hard of hearing and would smile and act like she understood us, even if she didn't! Yet she was a master "42" player and usually was on the winning team. Somewhere in the midst of these celebrations, our brother-in-law, Jack Boggs, would say "This is *really living.*" We knew he was right. It was. It would be the strong family bonds and wonderful memories, built layer-upon-layer, which would carry us through the most difficult times of our life that we could not yet see, even though they were on the horizon. As I reflect on this, it was such a work of God's grace. In His providence and sovereignty, He of course knew what was coming. He met so many of our needs long before they came. The words of my mother from my childhood resonate in my soul as I write this: "Sonny, we may not have much, but we are *rich* in what really counts."

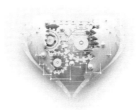

2001

Life was not perfect as we moved into 2001, but our afflictions were "normal." Mary was dealing with severe back pain that came from scoliosis, which we discovered only at this point that she had had all her life. I seemed to have constant knee pain as I limped around trying to "tough it out." Rachel was struggling trying to figure out if a long distance relationship had any future. We went into the year with these normal issues. Our lives would be forever changed by the time we began another year.

In early March, 2001, Rachel's relationship had ended and we knew that she was distressed and depressed, so Mary and I put everything in Denton on hold and flew to Washington to spend a couple of weeks with her. A very wise counselor explained to us the nature of the environment for young people like Rachel, who lived a stressful life on the "fast track" in the nation's capitol. The work was challenging, but the sense of competition and loneliness left many of them drained and distressed, exactly where Rachel was. We went to the animal shelter, and she found a cat that she named Jack. Having Jack meet her at the door of her apartment when she came in at night helped with the loneliness. We left believing that she was better, but knowing she was facing lots of challenges. We were thankful that she was involved in her church and in the midst of the challenges, still exhibited genuine faith.

Shortly after we returned to Texas, it was time for Dave to go to Milwaukee for the typical two months of six-day-a-week work on the Harley Davidson parts catalog. During this time, unbeknownst to us, he began having night sweats and his strength waned as the project progressed. By this time, he and DLynn had been married almost three years, and DLynn had to remain in Texas to teach. We heard very little from Dave during this time, attributing it to the busy pace of the project.

Mary's back problem had reached a crisis point for her. In early April, Dr. Kevin Gill proposed that he do some surgery on her back to scrape some of the bone spurs and relieve some of the pressure on the nerves going through her diseased backbone. He did not give us a strong sense that this would fix everything for Mary, but that it should give her some pain relief and buy some time in the midst of everything that was going on with us. So he did the surgery. After a couple of days of hospitalization, Mary came home to recuperate for the balance of April and the early part of May.

While Mary recuperated, I had a challenge on another front. I was on the Board of Directors of Mission Possible Foundation, a ministry organization with ministries in Eastern Europe that had been based in Denton for many years. The decision had been made to move the administration of the ministry to the Chicago area, but the immediate on-going "maintenance" of the organization occupied much of my time. The financial times were challenging and some staff left and others were terminated. I was the only board member in the area. In this time of crisis, my involvement was critical to helping the organization survive. Two good friends, Gene Conyers and Dennis Dillon, agreed to do some part-time contract work to help get a handle on the books and the basic operation of the organization. In the late hours of the night, I went through the list of accounts payable and the bank statements in an effort to stabilize a downward spiral in the finances of the ministry. By God's grace, the ministry stayed afloat.

May was an important month in our family. Our niece, Libby Manning, was graduating from high school in the Amarillo, Texas area, over 300 miles from us. We made plans to attend and Rachel flew in from Washington to join us. Mary's brother came from his home in the Houston area and brought "Pop" to the big family event. Although Pop had lived with us for a couple of years, he had been with Mary's brother during the past few difficult months for us.

We arrived at the auditorium a little late, so I decided to let everyone out near the entrance since I would have to park a long way away. At this point in my life, I struggled with what seemed to me to be constant knee pain. As I began to try to reach the auditorium from where I parked, I could hardly make it. I stopped and sat to rest several times, and by the time I reached our family group, I was exhausted and soaking in sweat.

We had a nice time together. Mary's brother, Grover Royce, and his wife Anne, and Pop met us inside the auditorium. After the festivities of the weekend, our plan on Monday, Memorial Day, was that Rachel and I would fly from Amarillo to Dallas so she could connect to Washington D.C. and I could get back to work. That same day the plan was for Mary to start driving with her dad back home, stopping along the way at Wellington.

Rachel made it back to D.C., but I was struggling just to get through the airport. It gradually dawned on me that something more than my knee was afflicting me. I was short of breath and sweating profusely. I made it home and went to bed. When I woke up on Tuesday morning, I knew that something very bad was wrong. I decided to get in Mary's car and drive to the doctor's office. I noticed when I got in the car that my abdomen was swollen to the point that I could hardly get behind the wheel. I "blacked out" as I sat in the car in the driveway. In about half an hour, I came to and knew that I needed to get to the doctor's office. When I got to the doctor's office, without an appointment, I came in a side entrance and was seated in a back area until the doctor could see me. I was very "sleepy" and not alert to describe to anyone what had been happening, so I ended up waiting for a while. I was so "out of it" that I had no thought or capacity to try to call anyone in my family. When Dr. Bhatt finally looked at me, he immediately sent me to Denton Community Hospital, where I would end up being hospitalized for the rest of the week.

Meanwhile, Mary and her dad had been making the drive down Highway 287 in our Suburban. They stopped for coffee at the Dairy Queen in Clarendon. When Pop went to the restroom, he collapsed on the floor in an unconscious state, his eyes glazed over. A quick 911 call brought the Clarendon fire department and the paramedics revived him. Since he was familiar with the hospital in Wellington, he was taken there. Mary repeatedly called me but was worried that she never got an answer. She was having trouble and I was the one she wanted to talk to about what was happening with Pop.

So here we were, each in a crisis and not knowing where the other one was or what was going on. When Mary finally got to Wellington and Pop was situated in the hospital there, she called Dave and DLynn, as she thought Dave might have returned from Milwaukee. He had. So Dave and DLynn began the search to try to find me in Denton. After a couple of hours, they finally found me at Denton Community Hospital, and we were all able to know the extent of our family health crisis.

Tests showed that I had a blood clot in my leg. In fact, what was happening to me was the long ago predicted decline of my cardiomyopathy into heart failure. I had lots of fluid and, by now, an enlarged heart. I could hardly breathe. Mary was finally able to leave her dad and come to be with me. Although we were concerned, we did not fully grasp the seriousness of what was happening with me. In fact, when I finally was dismissed from the hospital about noon on Friday, I was determined to prepare a one-page report for the annual Mission Possible board meeting that afternoon at DFW airport. Mary drove me and helped me get to the meeting. God's grace saw me through the meeting and then back home.

I had two hospital stays at Baylor Medical in Dallas over the next six weeks. My medication was changed, but the slow, methodical grip of heart failure had taken a toll, and I constantly had trouble with energy and breathing. For several more years I would mistakenly attribute the difficulty in walking to my bad knees, when, in reality, it was the continuing decline of my heart capacity.

In the midst of all this, Dave and DLynn came by one day to visit. They shared that DLynn was pregnant and that we were going to be grandparents in February! We rejoiced at the wonderful news.

In late June, we all four went to the grand opening of our friend John Duncan's scan clinic in the Las Colinas area. There were refreshments, a ribbon cutting, and then a drawing. The prize was a free body scan. Dave won the prize and soon went back to Las Colinas to have the scan.

In July, Mary and I decided that we needed a little break and a chance to reflect on our circumstances, so we spent a few days in Red River, New Mexico. On the way back to Denton, we stopped in Floydada, Texas, to see my mother and sister. At a restaurant in Floydada, we had an unusual encounter with a stranger who approached me and asked to pray for me and my health (my struggle was obvious) and, as he said, for "the old lady, as she doesn't have long to live." He prayed. It was the third week of July.

Mary talked to David on the cell phone and was alarmed to hear for the first time about the challenge of the night sweats. He had been to our family doctor, Don Holt, who told him he might have tuberculosis. The results from the scan that had been done at John Duncan's office suggested that something was wrong.

Our arrival in Denton commenced a series of intense appointments and efforts to get a good diagnosis for David. A biopsy was scheduled at Denton Regional Hospital. He had severe back pain and we realized he might have a serious disease. The guess was Hodgkin's lymphoma, but it would need to be confirmed by the biopsy, which was very slow in coming. We called our pastor and a group surrounded Dave and prayed for him in the chapel at Denton Regional on the day of the biopsy.

We were referred to a cancer specialist, Dr. Claude Denham at Baylor Medical in Dallas. Interestingly, almost a decade before he had treated Dave's second cousin, Tim Cypert, who had survived virtually the same illness. Our appointment was scheduled for Monday, August 13, 2001. That day would be our thirty-fourth wedding anniversary.

The day before, Sunday, August 12, 2001, my sister Molly called from Floydada to report that mother had had a slight stroke and was in the hospital at Lockney. She thought she would be okay after a few days in the hospital.

Our family drove to Dallas quietly on Monday, August 13. I prayed in my thought-life that this would all get cleared up quickly and soon everything would be back to normal. Most likely all four of us, Dave, DLynn, Mary, and I, were having the same thoughts. We just did not open up and voice them. Dr. Denham was a quiet soft-spoken man, and that added to the pensiveness of the day. Although the situation pointed to Hodgkin's disease, without a good biopsy it was not certain. Dr. Denham ordered another biopsy by a Baylor surgeon, and expressed that in a follow-up appointment, he would also do a test of the bone marrow by using a large needle to draw marrow from Dave's back. I flinched as I thought about it. Dave was a husky and healthy man, but he had always had an aversion to needles and blood.

My thoughts drifted to the time when he was a senior in high school, really enjoying life before graduation. He received the word that he did not have enough service hours to get to wear the "tassel" for the National Honor Society in the graduation ceremony. He was given the last-minute option of donating blood to fulfill the service requirement. So I agreed to go with him to the old Westgate Hospital in Denton so he could donate blood. I had been a blood donor for many years, so I did not suspect that this would be difficult for Dave. It was not difficult … after hours of coaxing and waning courage, it was impossible. I don't know how he managed it, but he did walk in the ceremony with the tassel. He was not able to bring himself to donate blood. In the years that would follow, he would undergo some of the most painful treatment with needles, IVs, and ports. God gave him courage and grace, and he endured.

By the time we left the appointment, we were all frustrated at the slow pace of getting a diagnosis with such a mortifying possibility looming.

The next morning, my sister, Molly, called early and told us that somehow it seemed that mother was going downhill and might not survive. She had told Molly that she would really like to see all of her children. Mary and I methodically packed our things in order to make the five-hour drive. Given our sister's ominous assessment, we packed our best clothes so that we would be prepared for a funeral. Molly said that our sister, Jo Boggs, who lived in Yuma, Colorado, was leaving to drive to Lockney, where mother was hospitalized. We realized it would be late in the day when Jo arrived, so we lingered in Denton after we packed to go by and see Dave and DLynn. While we had all the awful thoughts about Dave's health, we still had that inner joy of knowing that our granddaughter Tatum was being nurtured in her mother's womb. We enjoyed seeing them just to get a sense of that miracle!

Very late that afternoon, all of us—my brother, Wes, and Wynelle, his wife, our sister, Jo, from Colorado (Jack couldn't come that quickly), Molly and her husband Bill, and Mary and me—were all gathered around the bed of our mother at the Mangold Hospital in Lockney, Texas. Molly had been an RN at this hospital for many years, so this was a close, intimate family time among friends. There were no interruptions. During the day mother had shared a number of things that Molly had written down. Molly shared all those with us, and we joined hands and sang songs and prayed together—time seemed to stand still, and mother seemed so bright and alert. She enjoyed the time immensely. It was only weeks before that the stranger at the restaurant had prayed for her and said, "She doesn't have long." Molly told us how, when the first news that Dave might have Hodgkin's disease came to Mother two weeks before, that she just went and lay on her bed and did not get up. God had determined that she had had enough battles in her eighty-six years, and that the long one ahead was not to be hers. Yet the grit with which she lived would continue in the generations to come. She died quietly and without pain the next morning in the presence of my brother and sisters.

Mother was the last of a whole generation. Our father was the youngest of twelve children, so when mother died at the age of eighty-six, she was by age and attitude and outlook, the dear matriarch of our entire family on my father's side. This would be an occasion rich with joyful memories, as many family and friends began to gather from all directions for her funeral service which was on Friday, August 17, 2001, at the First Baptist Church of Floydada, Texas. Dave and DLynn came. Rachel flew from Washington, D.C., so all Opal's grandchildren were present. Grandsons and grandsons-in-law served as pallbearers. There was much sharing and music during a very long and memorable funeral service that I conducted. She was compared to the shade of a giant tree that covered all those under her with protection. After the service in Floydada, our family hurried to get on to Knox City, about a two hour drive, for the burial next to our father, Joe Earp. Many family and friends from Knox county and Gillespie Baptist Church gathered around the graveside as we celebrated her life again.

Back home we were in a hurry-up mode to get to the truth of David's diagnosis. I went with him to meet with the surgeon at Baylor who would do another biopsy. By now DLynn was busy back at school, so we coordinated our schedules to deal with all the back and forth to Baylor. DLynn was with Dave the day of the big needle in the back at Dr. Denham's office. It was one of the worst from what would be eventually be a five-year ordeal. Literally an effort was made to pound the needle into the back bone to get bone marrow. After much agony and repeated tries, Dr. Denham could not get any bone marrow. This was not a good sign.

And then came September 11, 2001, which forever changed the course of history. Mary and I were following our normal routine of breakfast and then our devotional reading from *Our Daily*

Bread. The minute we turned on the television, we were drawn into an entire day of watching and waiting in disbelief. Fear and anxiety swept over us. We watched the destruction of the sense of security we had always felt evaporate before our eyes as first one and then the second of the World Trade towers were hit by terrorist controlled airplanes. As the news unfolded, we realized that we would never be the same after this day.

Then the report came that another airplane had hit the Pentagon. Fear for Rachel immediately consumed us. Although her office was a few blocks from the Pentagon, she was often in the Pentagon for meetings that lasted all day. We immediately began to dial every number that we had for her, without any answer. The routine for our day was set. I would dial. I would then report to Mary that there was no response. We were in constant prayer. We said to each other dozens of times, "What has happened to her?"

Her office was a secure facility, and finally by mid afternoon I was able to reach one of the guards at the guard station. He assured me that the building had been evacuated and he was sure that he had seen Rachel (her long blonde hair is hard to miss) hurrying out the door. At last we felt some relief! Later that night David was finally able to get through to Rachel and talked to her for a few minutes. She had quickly traveled the two miles to her apartment and sequestered herself, waiting for any official communication from her work associates in the Department of Defense. The previous afternoon she had been in a long meeting in the very area of the Pentagon hit by the terrorist attack. When the dust had settled from this terrible day, eight of Rachel's peers would be counted among the dead. There would forever be the shadow of fear and death as September 11, 2001, changed everything.

The event of September 11 is a picture of the destructive and devastating events that came to our family in 2001 and continue even to this day. I have many investment clients, and the events of 9/11 and the subsequent crash of the financial markets added a layer of distress to our lives. For a short while, it seemed that panic might prevail, but then strength seemed to emerge, along with a determination to counter the impact of the terrorist attacks. In many ways, that paralleled the personal battles that had begun in our lives.

Finally the diagnosis came in that David had stage-four Hodgkin's disease. Only later did we have an understanding of what that meant. A respected doctor told us, sometime later, that stage-four Hodgkin's had long been considered a "death sentence." We were oblivious to that, praying and hoping for the success of several months of chemotherapy.

The early part of the chemotherapy was tolerable for Dave. DLynn drove with him for the treatments when she could, but more often, Mary and I would take him. We now know that this initial chemo had little chance to eliminate the advanced stage of Hodgkin's that he had. The infusion room on the second floor of Collins Hospital at Baylor had many cubicle-like spaces. In each space there was a reclining chair where the patient sat and then reclined. There was a small TV just overhead. A nurse would come in with a bag of drugs, hang them on an IV pole, and then hook Dave up. His needle phobia from childhood became a distant memory. Some days, there was not much immediate impact. On other days, he would throw up in the car on the way home.

David's emotions were buoyed by the anticipation of the birth of Tatum Grace Earp. Although we worried and prayed, our whole family rejoiced in the development of this first grandchild who would come into our family.

We had one unexpected moment that autumn that would have an impact on Dave's future treatment. We invited Don and Linda Carter to lunch one day after church. They are well known in Texas for their business acumen and philanthropy. They had moved to a place north of Denton and had joined our Bible class. It was normal for Dave and DLynn to tag along when we had lunch after church, so they joined us. During the course of our conversation over lunch, we talked about the treatment that Dave was getting at Baylor. Linda shared with us that she had a sister who was a cancer survivor and who had been treated at Baylor. As we were leaving, Linda Carter whispered to Mary that the next year, she would be President of the Board of Directors of the Baylor Medical System, and if in the course of David's treatment he needed anything, to call her. During the next few years, we would feel the shadow of Linda's influence in many positive ways.

We had enjoyed Pop living with us for the past couple of years. He had regained strength and his health was better. Either Mary or I would take him to the Senior Citizens' center most afternoons, where he would play dominos with some friends he had made there. But now with David's challenge, the situation with Pop had changed. Pop made the transition to a residential care facility in his old home town of Wellington. A close friend, Connie Dwyer, who had been Mary's mother's hospice nurse, had opened this facility. He enjoyed being back in Collingsworth County and having old friends and relatives stop by for a visit. In November, he was hospitalized at the Collingsworth County Hospital, and we drove the 240 miles quickly to be with him. When we arrived, we were alarmed to discover that he was in isolation. For a couple of days we wondered if he would survive. Somehow he recovered. Once again he had lived up to his "Energizer Bunny" reputation. This would become a familiar trip that we made many times as he was in and out of the hospital over the next year and a half.

I struggled with my own health during this time, but I focused on bearing up and being there for my family. The joy of having a grandchild masked many negative issues in our life.

One day as Dave sat in a chemo chair, a group of nurses with balloons and an air of excitement celebrated with a patient just a few yards away who had completed chemo and been pronounced "cancer free." Such a celebration buoyed our hope that Dave's chemo treatment would have the same outcome. With the chemo finished, we enjoyed Christmas. Rachel flew in for the holidays. This was the first of many Christmas times that had a darkness that threatened to cover the truth of why we celebrate. We moved into the year 2002, still hoping that prayers would be answered, David would be cancer free, and we would emerge from all of these challenges unscathed.

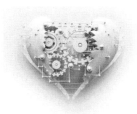

2002

David was assisting in some photography shoots in the Fair Park area of Dallas on some days in early 2002. This was close to Baylor, and on one of those days, he had a scan to check the outcome of the chemotherapy.

Can one day be any better and the next day be any worse? That is the only way to describe February 25 and 26, 2002. DLynn went into labor early on February 25 and headed to Community Hospital. Dave hurried to finish a deadline and then met us all at the hospital. Before noon, Tatum had arrived. DLynn had a normal delivery, and Tatum was a healthy eight pounds. Dave was with DLynn during the delivery and they shared the ecstatic moment of her birth. Mary and I stood outside the door and listened for her cry. We were joyful grandparents! Soon Dave appeared at the door beaming, holding Tatum in his arms. We watched as the nurse carefully bathed her and held her up for us to see through the glass of the nursery. We had many family and friends who joined us in "ooing" and "ahhing" as we watched Tatum in her early hours. Soon DLynn was in a regular room. What a blessing it was when they brought Tatum in to her and Dave held her, and then we had a chance to hold her, too! It was such a euphoric day.

We had made it our practice to be with David on visits to Dr. Denham in Dallas as a matter of support and encouragement. In the excitement of Tatum's birth, it escaped us that early the next morning Dave went to Dallas to Baylor by himself to get the results of the scan. By noon he was back to the hospital, and by the expression on his face, we immediately knew that something was very wrong. He blurted out the news. The cancer was not gone, but had spread. He would be turned over to the Bone Marrow Transplant Center at Baylor. It was such awful news. We called some family and friends, and soon our pastor and lots of people were with us. The waiting room at the hospital filled with people as the news spread. Many people had already been praying for Dave. Now a more urgent and intense prayer-time began.

In the middle of March, our whole family, including Rachel, who flew in from D.C., went to Dallas for the initial consultation at the Bone Marrow Transplant clinic. This group was located on the first floor of Collins Hospital. There were five doctors in this unit. We would become well-acquainted with all five of these doctors. Dr. Luis Pinero was Dave's primary doctor. As we waited around the table, a Baylor chaplain, Reverend Travis Maxwell joined us. Then others from the Baylor Foundation came in and introduced themselves and stayed with us for the duration of the meeting: They were surely shadows of Linda Carter's commitment to help. We liked Dr. Pinero and his nurse, Tamara. We immediately came to appreciate the social worker, Phyllis Yount. The whole staff became our friends.

A different type of chemo was described, but Dr. Piniero told us that it was likely that Dave would have to have a radical, high-dose chemo. As we were heading home, Dave got a call from his photographer friend, Mark Harmer, and they discussed the possibility of Dave's being involved in the Harley Davidson parts catalog shoot in Milwaukee in April and May. Clearly this was something that Dave wanted to do.

The Harley shoot was, in fact, a two month photography marathon, as the team worked six days a week, sometimes ten hours a day. Dave loved the camaraderie with his old associates at Midcoast studios. But physically, it was no cakewalk. Dave was battling cancer and needed treatment.

Some things were in Dave's favor to do this. DLynn was on maternity leave for the rest of the semester, so she and Tatum could go with Dave. The crew always stayed at a nice Hampton Inn near the shooting site, so there were good accommodations for DLynn and Tatum. And Dave's charm came through to Dr. Pinero and Tamara. They could easily see his passion to be able to do this. During the next three months, the treatment regimen was another kind of chemo that would be taken weekly. The treatment was not available in Milwaukee. Finally, arrangements were made for the treatments to be done at a cancer clinic in Chicago, about 100 miles from Milwaukee. So, the plan was concocted: their little family would go to Milwaukee for the two-month project and one day a week they would drive to Chicago for Dave's chemo treatments. Dave's friends on the photography crew made the adjustments necessary for this arrangement to work. Mary and I were focused on battling the cancer and didn't agree that this project was a good idea. We kept this to ourselves. We realized that Dave had taken many emotional and physical hits, and could see that this might give him a needed boost and strength and encouragement for the big battle to come.

The time in Milwaukee had its challenges with a new baby, a long drive for chemo treatments, and the grind of the work. Meanwhile, Mary and I focused on our own issues. Her back problems persisted, and various doctors' appointments gradually brought to light the fact that her severe scoliosis was beginning to collapse her spine. She had constant pain and trouble with her feet, further indications of the sustained impact of arthritis on her spine and joints. It manifested as knee and foot pain in addition to the back pain. I struggled to walk and get around, but pretty much tried to bear up and do what I could for these others in my family who had more urgent problems.

We made a quick trip to Wellington to check on Pop. His health was fragile, but he liked the place where he lived, especially Connie, who pampered him.

We had a nice distraction of our own in May. Rachel completed the long-dreamed-of graduate degree from Georgetown University, so we flew to Washington to attend her graduation. We hosted a little party in her honor with some of her friends. Although she had carved a life out for herself there, we could see that she did not have passion for where she lived, and she was very concerned about the outcome of the severe cancer that her brother had. She and David were different in many ways, but after growing up only one grade apart, they were very close.

The Department of Defense began to help Rachel try to find a job opportunity in our area. In early June, she flew to Texas and she and I drove to San Antonio, where there was a possible position with Lackland "Security Hill." We spent part of the day looking at houses to try to give her a feel for what it would be like to live in San Antonio. But San Antonio was more than 300 miles from where we lived. She knew no one there. As we drove back, she realized such a move was not right for her.

By then Dave and DLynn were back from Milwaukee and started the planning process for the high-dose chemo treatments at Baylor. The Bone Marrow group had by now relocated to much better accommodations on the fifth floor of Collins hospital. During a couple of long appointments, we learned that the high-dose chemo would require a month of everyday treatment, much of it in the hospital. Arrangements were made for our family to have an apartment at the Twice Blessed House at the edge of the Baylor campus. By the first of July, we were moved into the apartment with Dave, DLynn, and Tatum. While DLynn was with Dave, Mary and I took care of Tatum in the apartment. When Dave could, he would return to the apartment. But he was sick, oh so sick, on-his-knees-in-the-parking-lot-throwing-up sick.

Before the high-dose chemo began, his stem cells were harvested and stored. A port, needed to handle the large volume of drugs that would be going into Dave, was surgically inserted in his upper abdomen just below his left shoulder by Dr. Capeheart. Then the application of the high-dose chemo began. It would need to bring him to the point of death. His white blood count would go to zero in this process. If and when he came back, the hope was that the cancer cells had been killed by all the drugs.

Meanwhile, Rachel's relocation plans were moving quickly so she could be nearby. She flew to Texas to complete the plans to accept a position as a Special Agent with the Inspector General's office and would be located in the FEMA, region-six building in Denton. She completed the paperwork to purchase a house only about ten minutes from where we lived! She spent some time with David, who was now hospitalized in the Bone Marrow Transplant floor, which was the fourth floor of Collins Hospital. Then she returned to D.C., anticipating moving in early August.

David's hospitalization during this July high-dose chemo time is a very memorable one to me. DLynn, Mary, and I rotated and kept a vigil. One of us stayed with David at all times. We had to be especially careful to wash our hands and use a mask so that the possibility of any infection was minimized. Gradually additional drugs were added to the chemo regimen. These were hung from an IV pole beside his bed. At one point, the number of IVs reached seventeen! The nurses called the IV pole with all its branches to handle seventeen IVs a "Christmas tree." The labyrinth of tubes and their plastic connections boggled my mind. The specially trained nurses would very carefully connect and reconnect the tubes as the IVs were changed. Occasionally one of them would have the task of following all the tubing and making reconnections to simplify the labyrinth. There was such complexity in this system of tubes and connections that Dave asked for his camera to take pictures of the "medical art work."

Dave had times when he was very sick, and then there would be moments when he was awake and lucid. My time with him was often in the middle of the night. Some of the most intimate conversations and prayer times in all our lives occurred during those times. Dave had always been an avid reader. We would discuss difficult topics like life and death and why cancer comes and why it came to him. We would read Scripture and cry. He especially loved the writings of Phillip Yancey, who wrote with great insight about the issues we discussed. Dave's personality and mine were very much alike in the area of mercy. So there were lots of tears. But there was laughter, too. Often the late-night nurses would sit and listen as we told war stories of funny things from the past and laughed and laughed. The strong drugs had their effect, and Dave's white blood count reached zero about three weeks after the process began. This was such a precarious time. It seemed that Dave was suspended between life and death.

The apartment had a television and a video player, and we became endeared by the experience of watching five-month-old Tatum laugh and enjoy the *Baby Einstein* videos. *Baby Galileo* had a panorama of color that her little eyes followed intently. She moved with the music of *Baby Mozart*. Tatum's isolated life in these close surroundings was such a contrast to what "normal" life usually is for a baby. A few blocks away, her daddy was holding onto life by a thread. Yet she thrived in the midst of the hush that covered our lives.

Every morning in the wee hours, a nurse would draw blood from Dave and, by 8 a.m., would write on a white board in Dave's room the various blood counts. Every time I entered the room, I would look to see if he had any white blood count. It seemed like the days when the white count was still zero were never ending.

Meanwhile, Rachel's moving-date was looming. We had hastily made plans that I would fly to D.C. and rent a truck and help her get loaded and then caravan with her as she drove her car and I drove the truck back to Texas. She had to be out of her apartment by noon on August 1, so the plan was that some friends would help her pack, and I would arrive on a flight on July 31. We would quickly load the truck and leave for Texas by the afternoon of August 1.

I did not want to leave David's side until he had a white blood count. I was euphoric the morning of July 30 to walk into his room and see that he had a white blood count! By the next morning, his white count was moving up quickly and it seemed the crisis had passed.

That morning Mary drove me a few blocks to the Adam's Mark hotel in downtown Dallas where there was a shuttle to the airport. It so happened that the Mary Kay convention had been going on in Dallas and I was on a shuttle-bus filled with Mary Kay ladies who were chattering away. I silently stared out the window, trying to catch my breath at the enormity of the burden that lay within my heart. Friends from our Bible class had offered to help Rachel make the move, but there had been a strong inner voice that said that I needed to do this. At this moment, even though the white blood count crisis had passed, I had no idea if David would live or die. These same thoughts occupied me as I caught the flight. "Who was I kidding? I could hardly walk and something physical such as carrying boxes made me short of breath. How was I going to help Rachel get this done?" Then I got some solace in thinking that just maybe she would have a whole army of friends who would be there to help.

She picked me up at National Airport and I immediately sensed the discouragement of her situation. When we arrived at her apartment, I saw why. It was a mess. No real packing had been done. Her friends were dropping by to take her out for ice cream! She was gracious and enjoyed saying farewell to them while I frantically packed boxes. Now I understood why this job was not meant to be left to friends. Rachel needed me. DLynn, Mary, and I had been with David every day. Rachel was the one other person closest to him, and being so far away, she had gotten lonely, afraid, and depressed, wondering what would happen to her brother. Soon we were both exhausted from the packing and decided that we had to rest. We were supposed to be loaded and drive to Wytheville, Virginia, by the next afternoon. I went to sleep on the little lime-green fold-out sleeper that we had bought years ago for $25 at the Salvation Army in Arlington, Virginia. It was not comfortable, but neither were all these circumstances of life.

I had made arrangements for the truck some distance from where Rachel lived because of the cost savings and the flexibility. Penske allowed us eight days until the truck was returned in Texas. The return date was important because the paperwork on her new house was moving slowly and she needed to close on her house before we could move her stuff in. We did not want to get to Texas and have to unload her stuff into storage and then move it again.

We got up at 6:30 a.m. and I joined hands with Rachel and we prayed for a miracle. She drove me to get the truck and then headed back to her apartment to continue packing. It was rush hour and it seemed like it took forever to get the truck back to her apartment. One friend did come to help. Rachel's apartment was on the fifth floor of a huge complex named The Arlington House in Shirlington, a community in Arlington. Loading the truck would involve taking her things out the door and down a long hall where there was an elevator, then down the elevator to the ground level and through the loading area to the dock where I parked the truck. The truck came with a four-wheeler, but I realized that we needed a dolly to easily move the items. So I used Rachel's car to drive to a nearby rental place and get a dolly. It would not fit into the trunk of her small, two-door Chevy Cavalier, so I managed to fit it in the backseat. By now it was 8:30 a.m. and I was in a panic. As I drove down "Four Mile Road" back to her apartment, I noticed that there were a host of men standing on the corner of Four Mile Road and Shirlington Drive. These men were day laborers standing and waiting for someone to stop and give them a chance to work. I quickly calculated my limited cash. I had $80 and wondered at the wisdom of stopping and getting a couple of helpers. I had used such help from the "Y corner" in Denton, but this was 1,500 miles from home. Did I dare take the chance? And if I did, how would I know who to choose? This was not yard work. It involved all of Rachel's possessions, some with lots of sentimental value because of the faraway places they came from.

In a moment I had pulled over and sensed that a large, black man named Thomas and a small, quiet man named Lewis were the ones to help. Thomas got in the front seat, and Lewis weaved his small, wiry body around the dolly in the backseat. As we drove to Rachel's apartment, I quickly explained the dilemma, the deadline, and what I could pay. They willingly agreed. We pulled in beside the truck, unloaded the dolly, and pulled the lift door up on the rental truck. It was 9 a.m. and we had three hours. We took the elevator to the fifth floor, where Rachel was packing feverishly. The heaviest items, such as the lime-green sleeper and some large boxes went on the four-wheeler and dolly first, and then my two helpers and I went down the hall to the elevator and pressed the down button. We waited and waited. A full five minutes passed. My panic shifted into a higher gear. How many more unanticipated things could we handle? Finally, the empty elevator arrived from the upper floors, and we packed the items onto the elevator and went down. After we unloaded the elevator, Thomas asked for my pocket knife, which he had seen me using, opened the knife, and reached it up into a small opening at the very top of the elevator door. Magically, the doors stayed open! As we reached the truck, I was telling the guys that I wanted the heavy items at the front of the truck and tied down with the rope that I had. By this time, I was already exhausted physically, covered with sweat in the summer heat and humidity and my steadily-worsening heart failure. Thomas noticed this and found a chair on the dock area and brought it to the rear of the truck. Then he said, "Mister, sit down! I have been working for a moving and storage company in Birmingham, Alabama, for six years and I know how to load a truck. You stay out of our way and my little buddy and I will get this truck loaded for you." Obviously Thomas knew how to get around slow elevators and load a truck. His smaller helper did not speak, but he worked quickly in concert with Thomas.

That day that had begun so full of panic is one of the most memorable days of my life. Never had a heartfelt prayer been answered so clearly. Rachel was amazed and could not believe that the truck was loaded and the apartment was clean on time! While she went to the apartment office to turn in her keys and complete paperwork to get her deposit back, I drove the truck with my two helpers back to the fateful corner. I wept as I drove, explaining to the two how that Rachel and I had prayed that morning for a miracle. I told them that they had been God's answer, His angels to help us on this day. I wanted to pray for them. Thomas shared that he needed prayer for his family with four children. He had moved to the area hoping for a better life for his family, but now there was no job and their money was all gone and he was struggling to feed his family. I wished that I could do more, but he was happy with his $40 because he often waited all day without any work. He was wondering if he should move his family back to Birmingham. Lewis explained that he was a Nicaraguan immigrant and that he so wished that he might have a wife. So I prayed for Thomas and his family and for Lewis to find a wife. They took their $40 each and were gone. But forever in my memories, I recall the grace of God on that hot August day, and the two special men that He had prepared to help us.

I met Rachel for lunch at the Olive Garden nearby. We finished our meal, and readied ourselves to hit the road. At this moment, a new crisis emerged. Rachel had been holding her breath about the progress of the paperwork for her home loan and had received a cell phone call that, due to a bad correction in the stock market, her account would not be sufficient for her down payment. We spent some time on the cell phone and got some reassurance that some flexibility was possible. Then we hit the road. I led the way, followed by Rachel and her cat, Jack, in her car, which was filled with the most fragile items. We went west on I-66 and before long, we were headed southwest on I-81. We spent the night in Wytheville. The next day we followed I-81 to its intersection with I-40 and drove west to Jackson, Tennessee, where Mary's second cousin, Andrea Woods, lived.

Andrea and her husband had lived about two miles north of I-40 for many years. As a result, she became intertwined in our lives, especially David's, as our family, at various times, drove back and forth to Detroit, Winston-Salem, or Washington D.C. Her hospitality in the midst of some long journeys was appreciated one more time.

We departed the next morning with the intention of making it home that night. However, we did not have smooth sailing. First we stopped for Rachel to visit her former pastor and his family, who now lived in Memphis. As we arrived at their house, Rachel locked her keys inside the car. So while she and her friends visited, I explored the options for dealing with the problem and finally called a locksmith. It was almost noon and we had only gone 80 miles of the 500 we needed to go. The truck had a governor, which meant we could not go the speed limit on the interstate. Construction delayed us further. After a late lunch, Rachel decided to lead the way, growing tired of the slow pace of the truck. We had worried about our cell phones losing their power, and as result, I was soon in another crisis. The truck just quit running, and I coasted to the shoulder of the interstate, frantic that my cell phone was so low. I tried over and over to start the truck, without success. As the phone was going out, I did get a quick message off to Rachel to come back; then the phone was dead. At this point, she was almost half an hour ahead of me. I sat at the side of the road, waiting for her to return so that we could use her cell phone to call for help. I contemplated all kinds of dreary thoughts in the meantime of having to unload the truck and reload it onto another one to get us to Texas. Finally, she retraced her steps and pulled up behind me. She gave me her cell phone and I started to dial the Penske roadside assistance number. I had an impression to try to start the truck one more time. It started! We were about halfway between Memphis and Little Rock in a remote place. I told Rachel to follow me and maybe we could get the truck to a place where we had better options. I eased onto the interstate amid the heavy traffic and the construction. To my surprise, I was able to pick up speed and the truck ran fine. We kept driving. I soon realized that in my previous efforts to go faster than the governor allowed, I had triggered a "shut down" mechanism of some kind. As long as I stayed under the governed speed limit, the truck ran flawlessly. Only two days after a day of unusual grace, another one was unfolding. We would not reach home today. We stopped in Texarkana on the Texas side of the line. It was Saturday night and we were back in Texas.

Now following I-30, the next morning we drove into Dallas to Baylor Medical. It was great to see David. He was much improved. Now that his blood count was coming up, if he continued to improve, we could move out of the apartment and bring him home by Tuesday. I was relieved later in the day to finally park the loaded truck in front of our home in Denton.

For many years, Mary and I wondered if our two children would end up living their lives thousands of miles distant from us. They had both experienced lots of the adventurous life they seemed to want to live as children. Now they were both back in Denton.

Every day seemed to unfold with new challenges. In the midst of the things going on to get David home, the deadline to unload the truck and return it loomed. We had until Friday morning. In the meantime, the paperwork to close Rachel's house was not done. Early on Thursday morning I went with her to the on-site office of the housing addition to try to get permission to unload her items into the garage of her new house. The lady at Woodhaven homes, the builder, insisted that it was not possible, given that the close was still days away. There were lots of reasons that they had never allowed such a thing and were not even open to discuss an exception. I drove the truck and backed it up to the garage of the new house just in case. I left it there, still praying that God would somehow spare us the energy and frustration of unloading and then reloading the truck.

I had to drive David back to Baylor later that morning. He was extremely weak and it was a scorching hot August day. He had his labs checked and saw Dr. Piniero. Every day was a day of hope for David. So far, so good. It was about 2 p.m. when we headed back to Denton.

It occurred to me as we were driving north on Stemmons Expressway, that we would soon pass right by the building where the home office of Woodhaven Homes was located. I told David that if he felt up to it, I would stop and see if I could find anyone who could help on the dilemma about Rachel's things in the truck. He assured me that he felt up to it, so I took the exit and pulled up to the building. I told him that I would leave the vehicle running so he would have air conditioning while he waited, but he insisted that he wanted to go in with me. Sensing that something interesting might happen, he said, "Dad, I would not want to miss this!"

We found the building directory for Woodhaven Homes. The mortgage unit was on the ground floor. We walked just a few steps down the hall and went into that department. Unfortunately, the loan officer handling Rachel's papers was not in. The only person in the office was the manager of the mortgage group. She heard a quick version of our story and immediately declared there was no possibility of doing anything. I asked where the office of the president of Woodhaven Homes was located, and she told me that it was on the fourth floor, but there was no use in going there as he was not in and no matter, there was nothing possible to be done.

I told her that we would go to his office anyway. So David and I trekked down the hall and took the elevator to the fourth floor. The upper-level executive office was plush. The receptionist eyed us suspiciously. I was in my shorts and had my usual limp. David was very pale and totally bald from the recent treatments. We were apparently not the usual visitors to the president's office. She said, "May I help you?" in a businesslike manner. I told her that we were there to see the president. She asked why. I simply replied that I had come to ask for mercy. She looked puzzled and said that he wasn't in. I asked who the ranking executive was who was present. She said that would be the national sales manager. I asked to speak with her. She again asked why. Again I said to ask for mercy. She made a call and soon a very stylishly dressed young woman appeared. When she saw us, she introduced herself and I asked if we could speak to her privately. She was very busy, she said, but, perhaps out of curiosity, she invited us into the adjacent conference room. She then said that the lady from the first floor had called to "warn" that we were on the way up. She quickly told us that Woodhaven corporate policy prevented moving any items into an unoccupied house, even the garage, which had not closed. She was sure that we understood the liability and that her hands were tied.

I asked since we were there if she was not even willing to hear our story. She said she was very busy, but she would listen if I made it quick. I told her our story in brief in less than five minutes, and then simply said, "I didn't come to complain; I just came to ask for mercy at the highest level of Woodhaven Homes." She looked at me and then at David, tears starting to roll down her cheeks. It was now about 3 in the afternoon. Then she said that she didn't think she could do anything, but she would make some phone calls and try, but warned us not to get our hopes up. I thanked her and David and I quickly left. I called Rachel on my cell phone and told her I didn't think we had any alternative, so would she start calling and see if she could find a storage place to unload the truck when we got back?

When we got to Denton, I dropped David off and went to meet Rachel at the model home of the Woodhaven subdivision where we could discuss our options. When we went in, we were met by the Woodhaven sales agent who said she had received a call from the corporate office to say they were considering my request for an exception to their rules, but that it was not likely. However, if they did agree, it would be under two conditions: Rachel would have to have the policy number of a homeowner's insurance policy and we would have to have a new lock on the door that went from the garage and into the house with a key that she could keep. She would be in the model home until 7 p.m. It was now 4:30 p.m. We had not even talked to anyone about a homeowner's policy. So, I told Rachel to keep calling about storage locations and I headed toward downtown Denton to the Farmer's Insurance agency, which was the only hope for a policy. I knew Rachel had her car insurance with Farmer's. The agency was still open when I arrived, but they clearly were ready to close and go home. As I was going in the door, Rachel called and said the call had just been received and mercy was going to be granted if we could meet the two conditions. I quickly explained to the person at the agency that a homeowner's policy number was needed dated today. She said she would get on the computer and try since Rachel did have a Farmer's auto policy. Fortunately I had my checkbook with me, and I wrote her a check and had a policy number by 5:45 p.m. As I drove toward the house, I began to call friends from the Bible class that I taught at church, asking if they could meet me at the location to help unload the truck.

I was not sure what we would do about the new door knob and lock. When I arrived back at the model home with a document showing the homeowner's policy number, the Woodhaven sales agent became instantly energized by what was happening. I told her that we had people on the way to unload the truck. She volunteered to go to a Lowe's nearby and get the needed door knob herself. So we drove just down the street where the truck had been backed up to the garage since early in the morning. She went through the house and pressed the automatic garage door opener. Friends were at that moment arriving, and the truck was open and the unloading began. By 6:45 p.m. the truck was unloaded into the garage, but there was a problem in getting the door knob switched out. A friend pulled out his tools and carefully looked at the directions. At just 7 p.m., the knob was finally in place, the garage door was lowered, the Woodhaven sales agent locked the door to the garage from the inside and kept the key as agreed. Mercy was complete.

I drove the truck to Lewisville to return it on time the next morning and Rachel drove my suburban with David as a passenger, so we could drive on to Baylor in Dallas after returning the truck. That day David would have the drive-line removed by Dr. Capehart. It was a quiet Friday morning. That morning, Mary was attending the funeral in Denton of Judy Reed, who had died just a few days before on the Bone Marrow Transplant floor at Baylor. We had often seen her family go in and out of ICU during David's hospitalization. In the quietness of the morning while Dr. Capehart worked on David, I reflected on the mystery of mercy. We had just experienced it. Another family had not. And in the days to come, we would find our prayers for mercy to not always be answered in the way that we wanted. What a mystery.

The rest of the month moved quickly. David regained strength and was buoyed with hope. DLynn went back to teaching. Rachel started her job, closed on her house, and officially moved in. Things were looking up and settling down.

In early September, Mary and I took David to have a PET scan, a ninety-minute-long process that was the only sure way to show the status of the cancer. We were hopeful that after the

ordeal of the summer, it would finally be gone. The appointment to review the scan with Dr. Piniero was scheduled for Friday, September 13. DLynn took off from school and we all went
to the meeting, including Tatum, in her baby carrier. From the
moment that Dr. Piniero came into the room, I knew something
was wrong. He was usually so personable and he and David
would banter back and forth jokingly. This day was different.
He was agitated and didn't make eye contact with any of us as
he began. We expected the PET scan to show the cancer was
gone. Instead, despite the ordeal of the summer, it had grown!
The words faded for me. There was mention of various things
to try … maybe radiation, maybe a donor stem cell transplant,
maybe even a "dual transplant"—a transplant with his own stem
cells followed by those of a donor. Things were going the wrong
direction.

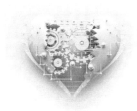

BATTLES

As we headed home, there was no talking. My mind drifted to another September day, 139 years before. I had not been there physically, but in my mind I was there at Antietam, the Civil War battleground near Sharpsburg, Maryland. That was the single bloodiest day of all wars in American history. From early in the morning, through the cornfield, down "Bloody Lane," across the bridge, there had been more than 26,000 casualties. I had visited that battlefield and tried to imagine the pain, heartache, agony, and misery. What I had heard about that battle was that throughout the night, the injured and maimed cried in agony from the carnage.

This September day in 2002 began our trip through the corn field, down "bloody lane"–our own unraveling experience of heartache, agony, and misery. We arrived in front of Dave and DLynn's house, now going through life's motions, fearing what was next. We hardly noticed it was a beautiful, sunshiny day. Mary found an old washtub and placed it on the front lawn. Then she lifted almost seven-month-old Tatum and placed her in the tub. She was dressed in white and as we looked at her toward the sun, the sunlight glowed around her. Dave got his camera and lay flat on the lawn and began to shoot pictures of Tatum. She reached with her soft, little hand to touch the blades of grass around the tub. The moment brought sunshine, the very light of God, into the misery and fear. Such, for us, would be the journey that would not last for moments, hours, days, weeks, or months, but for years and years.

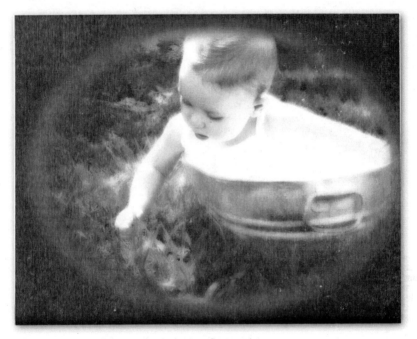

Tatum in the tub – September 13, 2002

Before September was over, Dave and DLynn had made a trip to the Fred Hutchison Cancer Center in Seattle, Washington. Mary and I kept Tatum, praying as we watched her crawl on the carpet on our den floor. Although the treatment program for Hodgkin's disease at Baylor in Dallas was well-known, the "Hutch" in Seattle drew patients from all over the world with the most serious cases of Hodgkin's disease. The doctors reviewed all of Dave's records and in a few days he and DLynn were back in Denton. The "Hutch" doctors spent only thirty minutes with him before telling him that they had nothing they could do for him. They gave him no hope or encouragement. Their view was Dave could try things that had been discussed in the uncomfortable meeting with Dr. Piniero just a couple of weeks before. The remaining days in Seattle, Dave and DLynn went to Victoria and Burchardt Gardens. Dave had left his pain medication home, thinking he would end up having some kind of hospitalization or treatment. His only pain relief came through some very potent drinks that DLynn arranged for him at the hotel. They returned to Denton, devastated by the prospects for the future.

We thought back in the summer that the high-dose chemo experience was the most withering treatment imaginable. We hadn't seen anything yet. Back at the apartment at Twice Blessed the months of October, November, December, and then January, 2003, passed with a blur.

First, there was a stem cell transplant with Dave's own stem cells. This was the first cycle of the "tandem," which they had never done at Baylor for Hodgkin's disease. In this cancer treatment setting, the oft used words "tandem" and "dual" are the same thing. A "tandem" is the cycle of first a patient's own stem cells, followed by weeks of total body radiation, and then a donor stem cell transplant. There were always battles. One was finding a donor. Another was getting the insurance company to agree to the tandem.

The strategy was to do the first transplant right away. It was done and Dave was out of the hospital and back to the apartment by Mary's birthday on October 3. That afternoon Mary and Dave had a cup of coffee at Café Brazil just by the apartment to celebrate her birthday. While Dave was recovering from the initial transplant, our friends at Baylor were working feverishly to try to get the second donor transplant approved by the insurance company.

Dave began the daily full-body radiation treatments. It was awful. He was so sick, again throwing up in the parking lot day after day as we drove back to the apartment. I had often heard the expression that the "cure was worse than the disease." As I reflect on it now, I am certain, in my mind, that the most physically devastating treatment for Dave was the total-body radiation. Life was methodical as we went to the first floor of Collins Hospital each day for these treatments. They were monotonous days with lots of dread and long times of waiting for the treatments. It was not just the nausea, or the endless waiting that were so upsetting. It was the hopeless looks of the patients who sat around us—the men without hair from the treatments and the ladies often with scarves wrapped around their heads. I was literally living in the "valley of the shadow of death." Death casts a shadow that hides any sunshine, and day after day we sat in that shadow, a pall over those around us. One day Dave confided to me that since he was a young man he had sensed that something bad was going to happen to him in his life. He was now experiencing the shadow that had come into his thought life years before. Anger and anguish welled in me. I suppressed expressing it, doing my best to be a calm loving presence in Dave's own agony.

Meanwhile, the search for a donor continued. The best match is a sibling, so Rachel tested to see if her stem cells were a match. They weren't. We learned that finding a donor was a difficult process. In order to be on the stem cell donor list, one had to have a blood test and be entered into a national data base. Not many people took the time and effort to do that. One of the reasons was that if there was a match, it was not just a minor inconvenience for the donor. Days of work had to be missed and medical regimens met.

By mid November, our prayers for a donor and for insurance approval were answered. The past month and a half had devastated David physically. On the day of his stem cell transplant, his body was bloated. He weighed a hundred pounds more than he had a year before. Every part of his body was puffy and with the absence of hair, he was a sight to behold. The awfulness of the treatment drained David, and it drained every one of us around him. DLynn tried to keep up with her classes, knowing there was a limit to the number of days she could miss without pay.

Tatum was a joyful distraction. Lots of family and friends pitched in to help with her. My two sisters came and stayed with her at Dave and DLynn's home. We returned to the house one day and they were enthusiastically saying to her "Chirp, chirp, Tatum Earp!" My memories are of her crawling around the Christmas tree in the cancer center, of her absorbed with *Baby Einstein* videos, and taking sound naps in the apartment as we rotated spending time with David. She seemed oblivious to the awful things happening to her daddy.

I was again spending deep nights with David on Collins' fourth floor and shuttling back and forth to the apartment. Our life was on hold. We were blessed to have family, friends, and a wonderful church. Without grace from God and help from them, we would not have made it.

We had always enjoyed the holidays in our family. During this ongoing battleground of our life, the holidays held no encouragement or joy. Dave tried to be home on Christmas day, but was so sick he was immediately hospitalized the next day. December faded into January, with our family rotating turns being by Dave's bedside.

In early January, Mary got a call that her dad had been taken to the hospital in Amarillo. There seemed to be some serious issues with Pop, so she took a taxi to the airport and flew to

Amarillo. Within a few hours, I was sitting beside David's bed on the phone with her as she called in a panic. The doctor who was supposed to be treating him was difficult and didn't want to interact with her or give her access to her father. He said that Pop didn't want any treatment. Mary knew of the distressed and sad condition that Pop was in and didn't believe he was in a stable frame of mind to make such a decision. I talked with the Baylor counselors who had helped us so much, and some ideas were suggested about what Mary might do. I called her and shared them. She followed the best suggestion and asked that the doctor be removed and requested the right for a medical review board to review his case. That happened the next day, and the board agreed with her. The doctor was removed, and Pop began to get treatment and improved.

By late January, Dave was improving and gaining some stability. While our family had not been given any encouragement that the devastating treatments would have any positive effect on David's outcome, we were relieved to have a window of time when we were not living in moment-to-moment crisis. By now we were out of the hospital, the apartment, and back home to Denton. Our regimen involved caring for Tatum, making every-other-day trips to Dallas to the cancer center, and trying to meet the minimum requirements of dealing with our own personal lives.

February was better, and by early in March, Dave had gained strength and was enjoying being at home. He had gotten accustomed to the medication regimen. We had been warned that never again would life be normal, but there would be a "new" normal. So there was a period of "new normal."

Meanwhile, Mary was back to regular trips to the Texas Panhandle as her father's decline continued. He had a tremendous capacity to bounce back from even the worst episodes. Then in late April we got the word that he was back in the hospital and made our way to Wellington. He seemed to be doing well enough in the hospital, but while no one was with him, he died on April 30, 2003. Our family was offered the mission house at First Baptist Church in Wellington; we stayed there while the arrangements were made for the funeral. FBC Wellington was without a pastor, although their long-term music minister, Derwin Comer, helped us with the details of the service. I ended up conducting the service. David was able to come with Wes and Wynelle. The church was almost full with family and friends. Rachel shared some moving thoughts about life on the farm with Memaw and Pop. Mary sang a beautiful song. David had creatively made a card that had a map of Collingsworth County with some recollections of Pop on the back. We buried Pop beside Memaw in the cemetery in Dodson. As the memorial at the cemetery concluded, the wind seemed to stir through the crowd, and then we saw a large roadrunner running by Pop's grave. It was a fitting end to a long journey.

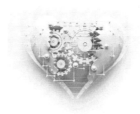

RESPITE

Although Dave had regular checkups and occasional bouts with nausea, "new normal" continued with him for a while. Mary and I were able to focus on our own situation. We had some great times in our Bible class as we were studying *The Purpose Driven Life* and having home groups. At one home group meeting, one of our group, Clint Knowles, approached me and told me that he intended to invite Rachel out on a date. I told him that would be fine, but to remember that she carried heat. Their first date was to the shooting range. When we had our patriotic party in June, Clint and Rachel were together, and Mary and I realized that their relationship was moving quickly.

Soon there was an engagement ring and plans for Rachel and Clint to be married at our church on October 11, 2003. Rachel's work situation required her to be in Louisiana often, so Mary dealt with many of the wedding details. Clint had worked many years with his family in the furniture business in Denton, so all of our close family lived nearby.

David planned the photography, and in a short three months, all the details were done. Mary had her moment as the mother of the bride. I rejoiced, escorting Rachel down the aisle. She was a lovely bride and we had a great time of rejoicing with our family and many friends. Clint and Rachel went on a wedding cruise and then started their life together at the house Rachel had bought when she moved back to Texas. It quickly became a home for the two of them.

During the darkest days of Dave's cancer treatment struggle, each day seemed like a year. But after Pop died, the time just flew by. The good days that we savored came and went, much too quickly. First the romance, and then the wedding, and then we enjoyed Thanksgiving and Christmas without a hospitalization! It was as if we went to sleep one night and had some good dreams, and then woke up. A year had passed.

Time stood still for us on a glorious, sunshiny Saturday on April 24, 2004. Mary worked as a volunteer for the "Relay for Life" a local American Cancer Society fundraiser at the University of North Texas Stadium. This day is always a celebration of life for cancer survivors, as they circle the track with their family and supporters. It was a great day for David. He looked better than he had looked in a long time. Tatum was two years and two months old. She had beautiful, curly blond hair that reflected the brightness of the sunshine. Dave reached down and picked her up and placed her on his shoulders, then began the trek around the track. Mary snapped a picture that we still treasure. DLynn and I watched from the stands as Dave circled the track. It was the high water mark in his cancer survival journey. It was a great day of respite in the storm and still gives me joy and energy when I reflect upon it.

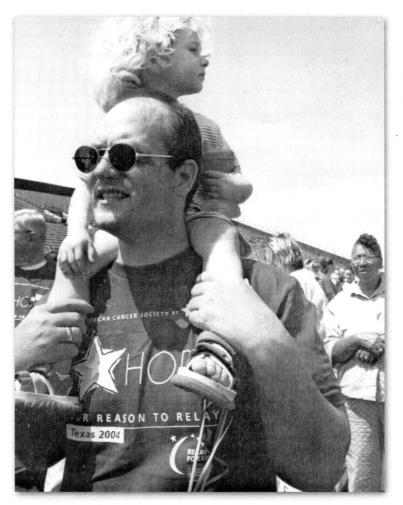

Dave and Tatum – Relay for Life, April, 2004

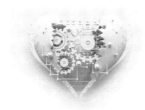

RISING STORMS

Mary lives at such a wonderful pace. When I think about her during these difficult years, I think about the phrase from an old hymn: "…when the storms of life are raging, stand by me…" Her faith was much like David's: not full of theological discussions, but a quiet, steady walk interspersed with questions and trust. I remarked to her one time about David that "if the soles of the boy's shoes were on fire, you would never know it." I could have said it about her, but I didn't. She just smiled, knowingly. Now Jesus was standing by her all the more. Her own pain and physical challenges had stayed on the backburner for far too long. One of her doctors convinced her that the bad pain in her foot and difficulty walking actually had to do with her spinal and joint issues. We knew the spinal issues couldn't be repaired surgically, but one thing that promised help was having her left knee replaced.

One of us was always having some kind of treatment, but this surgery required some serious time out. In June, 2004, she had the knee replacement surgery at St. Paul's Hospital in Dallas. Her knee surgeon, Dr. "Dicky" Jones, was known for how quickly he had patients up and walking after their surgery. She was walking the second day and came home the fourth day. His plan was not to have home health therapy; I had been to the classes with her and became her at-home therapist, doing the exercises with her several times a day. She progressed to using a cane, and was finally able to ride in the car. By the end of the summer, she was beginning to be normal.

As Mary gained mobility, I lost it. By September I believed that I could not make it any longer without having at least one of my knees replaced. I met with Dr. "Dicky" Jones and began moving toward knee replacement myself. I was very overweight and constantly sapped of energy. I was sure if I could just get one of my knees fixed, life would be better. I attended the classes and planned to get the knee replaced in November.

There was one hurdle in the planning process. Because of my heart history, I had to have a thorough heart checkup at Heart-Place at Baylor. I had been taking my heart medication, but with so much going on, I had not been to see Dr. Wheelan for a long time. I thought I was doing well and that this appointment in early November would be routine. Dr. Wheelan's physician's assistant hooked me up to do the Stress Echo on the treadmill. I explained to her that my knee was bad and that I would not be able to do well because of that.

I had done this procedure before, many times. First, you strip down and lay on the examining table on your back. Then the technician presses on a number of tabs all over your body, including your feet, so that wires can be attached to them. The wires attach to the stress echo device to give information about your heart as you begin to walk on the treadmill. Gradually the speed and the incline of the treadmill are increased and you walk as fast as you can as your heart rate increases. The readings are closely monitored and when you have gone as long as you can, you immediately lie down and turn on your side. Then the technician takes an ultrasound probe and applies a thick jelly-like substance to it and presses it against your chest in various places.

A nearby monitor shows what the heart pumping looks like. There is also the "swishing" sound of the heart pumping as the probe is moved to the various locations. The technologists at HeartPlace who do this procedure are very skilled and download all the data about the heart strength to electronic media for study and review.

Normally, the process is done in less than an hour and then you get dressed and wait a very long time. In a normal appointment, after a couple of hours of waiting, the doctor sees you and discusses the results. I have always been happy to leave. The waiting area is not a particularly pleasant place, with people of various ages all in some kind of heart decline. The process is often prolonged by an emergency. It is a sobering place. This is not "Heart Treatment 101." These are the people with the worst cases in a wide regional area.

On this November day, for some reason, they left me hooked up while the doctor went over the data again and again. Several doctors whispered back and forth in a series of medical huddles. As the afternoon faded into evening, my thoughts raced in all kinds of directions. All I wanted was knee replacement surgery to help with my mobility. Dr. Wheelan invited Mary to join us. Finally, he was ready to talk. I would not have knee surgery. At this moment, that became a very "back burner" issue. My heart capacity was declining quickly. He said my heart was so fragile that I would need surgery right away to install an ICD/ defibrillator.

Instead of knee replacement surgery before Thanksgiving, I had heart surgery. The decline of my heart capacity was so rapid I could almost feel it. My mobility likely was affected by my worn-out knees, but mostly it was due to the fact that I did not have enough blood flowing in my body. I lay in the hospital, sinking into a pit of sadness. I encouraged Mary to stay in

Denton for a day and spend some time with our family. I knew they were concerned and that she needed them. I just wanted to be alone. When Dr. Wheelan had shared the news of my bad decline, he had reminded me of the day almost fifteen years before, when he had said that if I lived to age sixty, it would be with a heart transplant.

God speaks in the most unlikely moments and in the most unlikely ways. As I write this, it is a cold, dark January day. Tears are welling up in me as I recall the sense of abandonment and desperation that I felt that November day. I remember being in the hospital bed, quietly drifting in and out of sleep with a mixture of sad thoughts and dreams. My friend, Matt Nelson, stopped by and sat in a chair beside me. Matt had his own history at Baylor, first as an employee–a CPA who did long-term financial analysis for Baylor building projects. And then he had his own personal challenges, some very tough times with his own cancer, and serious concerns for his family.

On this day, he simply sat by my bedside. Although he is a "talker" and in constant motion normally, he just sat quietly for a couple of hours. He asked if I was hungry. I showed him the menu and he called and ordered me a sandwich. Long into the afternoon he sat and read. Finally, he prayed with me quietly and was gone. A very quiet thought came to me. I remember the verse in Scripture where the Psalmist had said, "though I walk through the valley of the shadow of death, you are *with me*." I believed that God was with me. Matt's quiet presence beside me helped me hear the truth that no matter how hopeless I felt, God was with me. That moment would define what happened during the next four years.

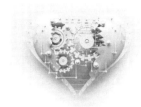

THE STORMS CONVERGE

I managed to make it through December with my friend, Gene Conyers, driving me on some appointments when I was not able to drive to myself. Then I had the black-out experience in my kitchen. At the beginning of this book I briefly described my initial appointment with Dr. Kuiper on January 7, 2005. I did not want to know about the LVAD, but I read the material anyway. I was quickly on some new drugs that had my head spinning. I went to the heart failure lab and took a medication that had to be given there. I was dying, and if nothing changed, I would be dead soon.

David's condition worsened. The side effects of the years of treatment were manifesting in a very painful way. He constantly had running sores on his legs and feet, which had to be dressed daily. He used some special support hose. In a particularly difficult moment I reminded him of the passage in James 5. This passage encourages the sick to call for the elders to come and anoint them with oil that they might be healed. I told him that the scripture said that the one who was sick should call for the elders. He asked and we discussed who the "elders" were. Our church has pastors and deacons, but not "elders." I shared my thought that from his perspective he should call those whom he trusted spiritually and who would pray in faith. So he called a few men - our pastor, Dr. Jeff Williams, and Dave's life-long friend Dr. Jim Mann, who is also a pastor in Denton, plus a few other men, including me. We met at Dave's house late one night. We prayed according to the scripture; I took the oil and bathed the sores on Dave's legs and feet in it. When we finished, I asked the gathered group if they would take the oil and anoint me and pray over me and my rapidly deteriorating heart. They did.

David was ever the determined one. The Harley Davidson Spring catalog shoot was coming up in Kerrville in late January and he was determined to go. I never wanted to discourage him, because these times and this work were important to him. It gave him a sense of professional purpose; he loved the guys he worked with, and his family needed the money. Things went well for a few days on the shoot and then David got worse. We drove DLynn to the airport to fly to San Antonio and Trudy Bastman, the art director on the shoot, met her and drove her to Kerrville. She brought David back to Denton. I felt so sorry for him. "Normal" was an increasingly evasive place in his life.

Meanwhile, I resolved to myself after reading the LVAD material that the LVAD was a dead-end street. There were no encouraging statistics. It just kept you alive. For what? More head-spinning and sitting in my chair, constantly dizzy, hardly able to move, listening to Mary cry in the bedroom. If I was going to go, then maybe I should be done with it and not try to hold onto a debilitated life, inflicting more suffering on my family. I went to see my pastor, Dr. Jeff Williams. He is surely my pastor and I love him. I had been the chairman of the personnel committee at our church when he was called to be our pastor. But he is a generation younger than me; it was sort of like talking to my own son. I knew I could not talk to David as I needed to talk to him. David's life was fragile, too. So I poured out my soul to the young pastor. I told him that I had decided not to do the

LVAD because it was a bridge to nowhere. He prayed with me and encouraged me by saying that he didn't believe that David and Rachel would want me to give up. I left reflecting on his wisdom but still resolved that the LVAD held no hope.

Our family has always placed a lot of emphasis on birthdays. Tatum's third birthday in February gave us a needed joyful focus. She was delightful and inspired her parents to get into a "Dave and DLynn project" with Grammy's help. Tatum wanted a playhouse that was big enough for her and her friends to play in. Dave and DLynn conspired and drew up some plans and Mary made a pattern, bought the fabric and the PVC for the framework and made it. It was huge. The party was held at the Denton Northlakes recreation center. The big playhouse was set up in the room, where the decorations contributed to a "Cinderella" theme. Tatum had a wonderful time. I labored just to come and sit quietly in the corner, my head constantly spinning with dizziness.

The next week a home-health nurse began bringing bags of a drug called debutermine that flowed intravenously into my heart. Mary turned again into a caretaker, changing the bags of medication and doing everything for me. As I sat in the chair in the den, with my head spinning, I prayed and I listened. I told God that I needed to know if it was His will that I die now. Our family had been through enough battles and I had already reached my personal conclusions about salvation and eternity. There was great assurance for me—no question. I based my convictions on what I believe to be the truth: that Jesus Christ in fact is the Savior who died for the sin of all mankind and that those who believe in Him and trust Him, though they die physically, yet will live with him in heaven eternally. I had wrestled with belief and I knew without a doubt that I did have a relationship with Him and that I would go to heaven. But when? So

I prayed repeatedly to know if this was the time, and I listened to hear an answer.

Honestly, dying seemed like it would be a relief from the endless swirling dizziness that I experienced every waking moment. There was no relief. I often found myself quietly pleading, "Jesus, help me." I knew that I was deep in the valley of the shadow of death, and I was ready to be in heaven. I agonize for you if you are reading this book and you are at such a place in your life, and you don't know Jesus. Who are you asking for help if not Jesus? The pages to come are almost more than I can bear to tell.

I now think of life using two metaphors: a journey that has stations along the way and also as a series of "life assignments." The stations ahead at this point in my life were like war zones, full of devastation and scattered debris. I asked God why these were my assignments. Why couldn't I get on the "good assignments" list? He has never answered my "why" questions, but, He has been with me. Along the way, He has helped me see that Jesus walked all the way through the valley, through the agony of the Garden of Gethsemane, and to the anguish of the capital punishment of the cross, and finally to the resurrection and heaven. Never would He take me anywhere that He had not already been.

In March I was hospitalized at Baylor twice and the ICD defibrillator shocked my heart back to life three times. Dr. Kuiper spent most of one morning with me in the heart lab. He ran a catheter through my neck and down into my heart, watching a monitor to check the condition of my heart. Heart failure is sometimes called "congestive heart failure." In the old days, it had been called an "enlarged" heart. In heart failure, the heart does become enlarged. As the muscle loses its pumping capacity, it works harder and harder to pump the blood, becoming enlarged in the process. When Dr. Kuiper concluded, he told me that my heart was the size of a small basketball. He could not remember seeing one that large, he said.

Back at home, I still had no clarity from God if it was His will for me to die now. Mary and I went to the attorney to be sure our legal paperwork was in order. I privately gave a list of the pallbearers for my funeral to a funeral director. If this was my time to die, I wanted to be ready spiritually for sure, but I also did not want to leave behind a mess for my wife. I completed a claim form on my life insurance and had it in an overnight envelope for Mary to send with my death certificate so that she would get the death benefit right away. I thought I would die soon.

Then one morning I was sitting in my chair, reading scriptures and I came to Psalms 27:13. The Word softly spoke to me. It simply said, "…you shall yet see the goodness of the Lord in the land of the *living*." I read it again and again. There stirred in me a conviction that God intended for me to live! By now my heart capacity was below 5 percent. I was almost bedfast, and my head was in such a whirl that I could not even sleep at night.

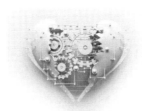

A DECISION TO HAVE THE LVAD

After sharing the verse with Mary, we decided to call Baylor HeartPlace and revisit the LVAD issue. Late in April, we met, for the first time, Dr. Daniel Marshall Meyer. Dr. Meyer is a distinguished Professor of Thoracic Surgery at Southwestern Medical Center in Dallas. He is the LVAD expert in our region, the only one who does this surgery in the major heart hospitals in the Dallas/Ft. Worth metroplex. He came to the heart failure clinic at Baylor to meet with us. We asked many questions.

The first question was obvious: what is an LVAD? I had originally only understood that it was some kind of artificial heart. I also had a vague idea from reading about it. An LVAD is very much like a water pump for a tractor from my days growing up on a West Texas farm. It is solid metal, very heavy, weighing almost five pounds. During the surgery, it would be placed in my body between my real heart and my stomach. It is attached to the bottom of the left ventricle of the real heart so that the blood can drop into it. On the other side of the pump it is attached to the aorta. As the blood drops into it, the LVAD pumps the blood mechanically up through the aorta to the rest of the body.

This mechanical pump cycles about 130,000 times a day pumping the blood. It is connected to a cable through an opening in the abdomen to a small square controller, a computer, about four inches square. It is designed to hang on the trouser belt. The controller is powered by two large batteries that are carried in holsters under each arm. At night, these batteries are replaced by a direct connection to a large (more than fifty pounds) power-base unit. There is enough cable, about seventeen feet, to allow some mobility while hooked up to the base unit. There are also six slots in this power base unit where the batteries are recharged. The two batteries last about three to four hours before having to be replaced by fresh ones. Since the LVAD is a mechanical pump, it needs a vent, which is located on the drive-line about eighteen inches from where the line emerges from the stomach. There is then another eighteen inches of drive-line to the computer/controller. As the LVAD pumps, there is a very audible "*swish*" sound that comes from the vent.

Since the blood is circulated by a mechanical pump, CPR is a non-effective technique. Thus the LVAD comes with a small manual pump with a bulb on it about the size of a tennis ball. This manual pump must be carried at all times, should the power or the LVAD fail. It has a hose that enables its attachment to the vent so that blood can be pumped with manual strokes on the pump.

Because it is a mechanical pump that has to pump twenty-four hours a day and seven days a week, it has a short life-span. It is not intended as an "end therapy," Dr. Meyer explained to us. We were talking about a bridge that would buy some time, maybe a year or two. My situation was so critical that we didn't even discuss what would happen after that.

Dr. Meyer answered all our questions. He did not offer glowing assurances of possible success. He was very direct. I didn't have any options. Finally he simply said, "Mr. Earp, I believe you need the LVAD, but you should do it soon." He didn't say "or else." We understood. My natural heart was virtually incapacitated.

Mary and I decided on the drive back to Denton that we should go forward with the process. This was a very difficult and costly surgery that needed preliminary approval from the insurance company. So we called back the next morning and requested that the process begin. And we asked everyone we knew to pray fervently.

In some ways I had lived these few months in a vacuum, even from my own family, except for Mary. They had all gathered on March 17 to celebrate my fifty-ninth birthday as if it would be my last.

There was, however, reason for celebration. Rachel was pregnant and due to deliver her first child in June. David had recovered from the spring shoot disaster and was well enough that he was planning to go do the Harley Davidson shoot in Milwaukee in April. His family needed the income. Tatum was now a delightful three-year-old and I loved hearing her call me "Grampsie." She was blossoming at the Children's Corner, where she spent most of her days. I realized that our kids and their families had their own lives to lead, so I had not really talked to them about the desperate struggle I had been going through. Only Mary really knew.

The paperwork process moved methodically along and the LVAD surgery was scheduled for May 17, 2005. Mary and I both tried to take care of last minute details. It was far too much for me to do, but I tried, leaving too many critical things hanging—a tax return that I just roughed out the night before with lots of notes, a lack of clarity about which bills had been paid and which hadn't. I realize now I was honestly incapable of doing what I had always done in our family and it left a scramble for Mary that has only been unraveled by the grace of God.

Our dear friends Jacob and Claudette Bernard wanted to fly in from Haiti and be with us and pray with us just the weekend before I had to go into the hospital on Monday morning. We had friends that thought it was too much for us to be entertaining visitors at such a difficult time. But it was a wonderful time, a time once again of quiet grace. Jacob and Claudette hovered by my chair praying quietly. As they were ready to leave, Jacob delayed coming down the stairs. When they were gone, Mary found that he had been upstairs cleaning the bathtub. We arose early the next morning, Mary packed the car, and she drove us to Baylor

I had almost waited too long. During the surgery, Dr. Kuiper later told me that the surgical team took off fifty-seven pounds of fluid, which my heart had no capacity to get rid of. A host of family and friends gathered to be with Mary and wait. After nine hours of surgery, I had to be returned to the operating room from ICU and have my incision reopened because of bleeding. I spent nine days in ICU where I also had a small stroke and some short-term memory loss. In all, I spent twenty-four days total in the hospital.

I have only a vague memory of coming to in ICU. There was great pain and I was instructed to click a morphine pump. The vertical incision ran the length of my torso. Large binder clips ran the length of the incision, holding it together. I could feel the vibration of the LVAD in my body and hear a constant *swishing* sound as it pumped my blood. There was another shorter horizontal incision across my stomach, and there was the hole in my stomach where the drive-line emerged.

SECTION II

LIVING WITH HEART #2

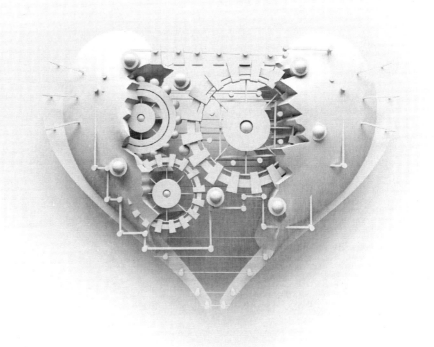

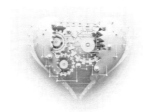

AM I REALLY ALIVE?

I had quite a new life in the ICU. You may recall the introduction to this book, which describes how I came to be the "Governor of Texas" in the ICU. With the morphine for pain and the lingering cloud of sometimes knowing what was happening, mostly I lived in a vivid world that was not real, at least to anyone else. But it was so real to me. There were a host of interwoven issues that swirled in my thought-life.

The ICU at Roberts hospital at Baylor is on the second floor of a seventeen-story high-rise hospital. Baylor is just on the east end of downtown Dallas. Another major hospital in Dallas is Medical City, located in the north part of the city, perhaps ten miles north of downtown. For some reason, it seemed to me that when the ICU nursing staff shift changed at seven in the evening, that one of the nurses would reach and push a switch on the wall. This would cause the second floor to hydraulically lift and gradually become the third floor. I could hear the sound of the hydraulic mechanism as it lifted. I worried that my family, who were only allowed to visit me for a brief ten minutes every four hours, would not be able to find me now that the ICU was on the third floor. One good thing about this arrangement was that when the ICU became the third floor, a back door opened from the ICU into a hallway that led directly into Medical City.

Not really. Medical City was ten miles away. But it surely seemed real to me.

The other thing that I gradually came to understand in my make-believe world was that the ICU was full of constant conspiracy. Many of the staff were plotting against me, and they were plotting against Dr. Kuiper. I can remember wondering if I should tell him that the ICU staff was out to get him. I believed that they were conspiring to kill me also. I dreaded certain nurses whom I believed to be part of the conspiracy to kill me. I would ask suspiciously what was in the shots that they were giving me. I was relieved if the shift changed and a "good" nurse came on. It was very clandestine. I did not want them to know that I was aware of their conspiracy. Fortunately for my family, my sister, Molly, is an RN and she clued into the imaginary, "ICU psychosis," world I was living in. So they played along. They started calling me "Governor" and worried with me over the constant plotting.

I worried that we would not be able to pay the hospital bill because our medical insurance was about to expire. I scribbled a note to Mary that it was very important for her to call an 800 number and "renew" our medical insurance. One particularly brave nurse sacrificed herself in the conspiracy to give me her personal bank account number and pin number so that Mary could "renew" the medical insurance. Not really. Yet almost five years later as I write this, I can visualize some of the digits in that bank account number the nurse gave me on the sly.

In the real and serious world of the ICU, three physical therapists came to my bedside to try to get me to stand up. They struggled time and again over several days. They told me over and over that to get out of ICU, I would have to be able to stand. I was too weak. Finally with a strap they buckled around me, they literally lifted me to my feet.

I felt suffocated by the ventilator. I got so tired of it. I was constantly hot and pleaded for cool air. Finally the staff rigged up a tube that blew cool air that I could blow on my face. This soothed me and helped me. By now, deep into the nine days I would spend in ICU, I was hungry and wanted the ventilator gone. My mouth was parched and dry. There were concerns about my lungs. Originally the thought had been that I might be on the ventilator and in ICU for four or five days. My real prayers were short and pleading. "Help me, Jesus," or "God, where are you?"

Finally on May 26, the concern about my lungs subsided. The ventilator was pulled, and I was moved to my new home on the Roberts hospital tenth floor heart unit.

The euphoria of being released from ICU increased as I was able to eat a Popsicle! I was still shaking off the effects of psychosis and realized that there was serious concern because I had had a stroke sometime during the process of being in ICU. I was examined by Dr. LaBeche, who began to ask me simple questions. Who was I? Where was I? What was the date? Then she asked me a simple math question: "How much is ninety-seven plus twenty?" Math had always been my strength. I could do it in my head, no problem. Not this time. I replied quickly "One hundred and seven?" Mary and my sister were in the room and immediately recognized my inability to do this simple math. Only later would I find out that night Mary had returned to Denton and confided to our family her concern that I might never really be "with it." Had the trauma of all that had happened to me resulted in a permanent incapacity? How difficult that must have been for her to wonder if my life had been preserved but not my mental capacity.

In the regular room I began to have visitors. My family stayed with me through the nights. David was back from the

Harley shoot. Rachel looked like she would deliver any minute. Friends sent cards, and a tie from our Bible class was clipped to the bulletin board. Rachel's last encouragement before her delivery was to bring some balloons and staple an impactful statement on the bulletin board. It was an old Chinese proverb that said: "A journey of a thousand miles begins with a single step."

I had yet to take the first step. In fact, my thoughts swirled, anxious about what was happening to my mind. What use was taking a step, or learning to maintain the LVAD, or hoping to go home physically, if there was no home to go to mentally? I pleaded with God, reminding Him that I had been ready to die, and He had been the One to preserve my life. Or had I misunderstood His signal somehow?

On the heart floor at Baylor, there is always a fast pace. This was my first of many hospitalizations on what I now call "Tenth floor Roberts." It would become a familiar place. Since it is ten stories up, it is near where the helicopters land as patients are brought from hospitals all over North Texas, southern Oklahoma, Arkansas, and Louisiana. From my room, I could hear the chopping noise of the helicopters land. This would be followed by EMT personnel pushing a stretcher down the hall to a room and lingering at the front desk, completing necessary paperwork. There were emergencies and alarming "code calls" all the time.

But there were a few constants. One was the process that took place early in the morning every day, beginning about 4:30. A technician would come in to draw blood, so that results were available when the doctors began their rounds as early as 6 a.m. By 5 a.m. a tech would roll a large scale into the room to get your weight. This was especially important with a heart failure patient, as the amount of fluid being retained in the body was an indication of the quality of the heart pumping function.

A DEFINING MOMENT OF LIFE

When the technician from the lab woke me to draw blood on Sunday, May 29, something seemed different. For the first time since my surgery twelve days before, my head was clear. For a few minutes after the technician left, I lay reflecting and listening in the quietness. I could hear the still small voice of God speaking in my thought-life. This was no illusion, hallucination, or dream. It was real. I felt joy welling up in me. My mind was clear and whole! I felt good. I knew in this moment that my life was preserved for a purpose. Quietly, I heard clearly that I was to write a book, I was to be a model and a leader for my family, and that I was to give myself to helping the poor and underprivileged. There were no flashing lights. I lay in bed, crying tears of joy.

Then Velma opened the door and pushed the scales in. Velma was one of the most constant things about tenth floor Roberts. For more than thirty years, long before Roberts Hospital had been built, she had been a tech working much the same as she did that morning. She had weighed thousands of heart patients in all her years. Her assignment today was difficult. I could barely stand with lots of help. So she summoned another tech to help get me up and onto the scales. Finally she read the electronic weight and wrote it down. The she began to take my blood pressure. I asked how much I weighed. She replied in kilograms. She finished and left the room. I was already trying to calculate in my mind how much my weight was in pounds, converted from kilograms. I made the conversion, certain that I was right. Later in the morning the first of my family to come to my room was my sister, Molly. When she came in, I said to her, "Sister, I am back!" I assured her that this was no make-believe kind of statement, that somehow that morning God had given me my mind back. I told her how I had mentally converted the weight from kilograms to pounds. Since she is an RN, she decided to go down to the nurses' station to see if my calculations were correct. The receptionist who always said "good morning" to all our family, Gladys, helped her and found the nurse to check the weight on my chart. Molly came back quickly and very excitedly told me that I was right!

This was a defining moment in my life. I did not know what the future held, but I did know that I was meant to be alive and make a difference. I got encouragement and energy to begin the long healing and rehabilitation journey. I still had not taken the first step, but I began to visualize myself traveling that thousand mile journey that would begin with a single step.

It was not easy, but with the cobwebs clear, we started back. "We" meant Mary and me. She had carried me to this point only by the grace of God. There was much for me to do, but much for her to do in adapting our life to living with an LVAD. The hole in my stomach that the LVAD drive-line came through was an open wound that had to have a sterile dressing change daily. This is a big deal. The first few times, Mary watched as the nurse did it. For me to live at home, she would have to learn to do this skillfully enough to keep the wound from getting infected. All the days that I lived with an LVAD, she was supposed to do this. The nurse demonstrated how to take the sterile kit and first clean my hospital room table that fit over my bed. Then she showed Mary how to "gown up," carefully putting on a sterile gown. There were two sets of gloves in the kit. The first was used in all the preliminary preparation–the "gowning up," the care in creating a sterile field on the table, the mixing of the solutions for the dressing change, and laying out the swabs to clean the site, and then the new dressing that would fit over the site after the cleaning. Then the first pair of gloves was changed, and the second set put on before the cleansing of the site. We learned that many of the failed LVAD experiences that led to death were due to infections in this open wound in the stomach. Once the site was cleaned and dressed, then all the materials had to be collected and discarded. We began to question how we would ever be able to do this at home. It gradually dawned on us that it would take a ton of supplies to maintain the LVAD and dress the wound.

Another issue was trying to learn how practically to use the LVAD, maintain the batteries and be prepared for emergencies. This was not some appliance that could go out and be replaced in a few days. It was pumping my blood! What if the power failed? What if the pump quit? How would I know if it was working correctly? What did all the lights on the computer mean? We learned that there were amber alarms and then there was a red alarm. We learned that we did not want to have a red alarm. I learned how to adjust the mode of the LVAD from fixed to auto or automatic. In fixed mode, the pump pumped exactly fifty times per minute. This was a minimal number of cycles that would assure a minimum supply of blood to the brain. When on fixed mode, I would get light headed since I was not getting all the blood supply I needed. The benefit of the fixed mode is that it takes less power. So if I happened to get into some type of battery crisis, I could change to fixed mode to prolong the life of the batteries.

The normal mode–"auto" allows the LVAD to pump the amount of blood that the body needs. So if I was just resting, it might do sixty or seventy cycles a minute. But if I started to do some activity, it would automatically cycle up to the number of cycles needed. The fastest rate that the LVAD had was 120 cycles per minute. That is really fast! Imagine a five-pound metal pump pumping inside the abdomen 120 times a minute. At this rate my insides literally shook and sometimes my teeth would chatter.

My head had just gotten clear and I had to learn all this. The advantage of being in a hospital bed all the time was that the drive-line was hooked directly to the big base unit on a cart at my bedside. On the seventeen foot "tether" I did not have to worry about batteries, and since I couldn't walk, the seventeen feet was plenty. But I practiced the process of switching to the batteries. The batteries were large, about two inches wide and six inches long. They fit into plastic clips which had the connectors to attach to the drive-line. Two batteries at a time were needed. They came with a "holster"–pockets attached to a black harness that fit around my shoulders so that the big batteries fit under my armpits. Over the next few days, I had repeated this process over and over. Gradually Mary and I began to get the hang of what we had to do to keep this thing going and keep from getting infected.

Then we practiced using the manual pump. The first emphasis in the training of the use of the manual pump was to always have it with you. We heard all the horror stories of someone forgetting their manual pump and having something fail with the LVAD. If the LVAD quits pumping for any reason, we learned how to take the manual pump and attach it to the vent in the drive-line, clear it, and then begin to manually pump the blood, squeezing two handles together manually to do the pumping. As a precaution, the instructions for using the manual pump were laminated to it.

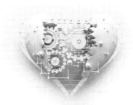

A NEW GRANDCHILD

By the end of the week, we were getting pretty adept operating and maintaining the LVAD. Then it was time-out for Mary as she was back in Denton when Rachel delivered A. J. (for Allen James–the names of his two grandfathers) on June 2, 2005. Everyone in our family was there for the delivery, except me. Rachel was doing well after the delivery, so everything in Denton was great.

I still was faced with a big hurdle: I had not walked. It had now been twenty days since I came to the hospital. The faithful physical therapists kept coming every day. I could stand and finally managed, hanging onto them and with them holding the strap wrapped around me, to make it to the door of the room. So far, all the physical therapists had been female and though they were adept at doing what they did, their small bodies were not strong enough to support my "eighteen-wheeler" bulk. I was now wishing to be home, but I could not go until I had walked at least with a walker a full two laps around the tenth floor, which was a long way!

Then Willie Lafitte appeared at my doorway. What a physical specimen Willie was. I learned that Willie was the "go-to" physical therapist for guys my size. He still looked as fit as he surely did when he was a Special Forces master sergeant. He looked at me and said, "Mr. Earp, we are going to walk today." Willie heard nothing of my complaints, excuses, or sad stories. He had the belt around me and me on my feet all the way to the door with me saying, "I can't." He placed my hands on the handles of the walker and my sister pushed a wheelchair behind me, and we walked, just a few steps, to the end of the hall. Willie came back later in the day and again we walked to the end of the hall. I began to sense going home was possible. It would not have been possible without Willie and countless others: young nurses, technicians, therapists, ICU staff who had worked diligently to see me through, and my family—especially my precious Mary. By God's grace, the very one who had said He would be with me, and that I would see His Goodness in the land of the living, we had almost walked through this valley of death.

There was just one more walk. I had to do the two laps around tenth floor of Roberts. This was scheduled for Wednesday, June 9. Mary was there. The "front row" was there, and three-year-old Tatum was there, her blond curls bouncing energetically. I made one circle and rested, trying to preserve my strength to do the last lap. I was hanging on with all my life, slowly coming around the last lap when I looked up and saw Tatum. She was about ten feet in front of me, facing me and walking backward. She was beckoning at me with her arms and yelling, "Come on, Grampsie, you can do it." I did.

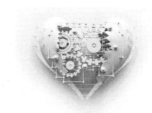

COMING HOME

We were amazed to learn that when we left the hospital to come home after getting the LVAD, that Dr. Kuiper and a nurse would come home with us! Our first stop was at the emergency room of our local hospital where the entire ER staff had been gathered for a training session on the LVAD and what they were to do if I showed up in their ER with my LVAD. Dr. Kuiper conducted this session, introducing me, and then demonstrating how the manual pump worked. There were many questions, and we left with some reassurance that the ER would be clued-in if we had a severe emergency.

Our next stop was the fire station nearest our house. Again, all the EMTs had been gathered, and again Dr. Kuiper explained about the LVAD and how they were to deal with it if they got a 911 call to come to our house.

Finally, we got to our house and Dr. Kuiper and the nurse came in and looked over all the arrangements Mary had made. We got the LVAD base unit plugged in and they were satisfied that the electrical modifications had been made and that everything was working correctly. Then they explained to us that on their way back to Dallas, they were scheduled to stop at the City of Denton Utility Department, where paperwork would be put on file, indicating that in the event of an electrical outage, the need for power at our house due to the LVAD was to be of highest priority. We were so encouraged at the level of preparation that had been made in advance to deal with possible emergencies!

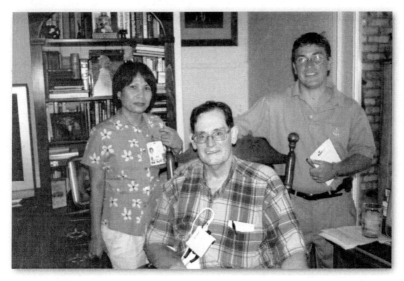

Exhausted Governor is home with the LVAD, with Dr. Kuiper and nurse

When we came home, we came with the basic equipment: the power base unit, a monitor, which shows the status of the pump when attached to the LVAD power base unit, a supply of twelve batteries, a manual pump, and a very heavy emergency twenty-four-hour battery in case of extended power failure. Central Supply at Baylor loaded our Suburban with boxes and boxes of the sterile supply dressing-change material, the gowns, gloves, and everything we would need.

Mary prepared for my coming home by having some modifications made to our bedroom. She had an electrician come and install a plug near our bed and properly ground it for the LVAD power base unit.

My family has a great way of making some kind of statement on a significant day. This day, it would be A.J.'s turn. Rachel came and placed A.J. on my lap. I was still seated in the chair that I had collapsed into when Dr. Kuiper came in the house with me. As I rejoiced to look into A.J.'s face for the first time, he made a statement—he wet on me! I was home.

I determined to go to church on Father's Day, June 20. David wheeled me in my wheelchair up to the worship center. What a joyous occasion this was. Our pastor allowed me to share a short word from my wheelchair and many people came by to greet me and our family.

The day-to-day was challenging. I needed to walk with the walker on my back driveway. The "front row" had helped in so many ways. I was the "baby brother" and my sisters had hovered over me in the hospital. Now my brother came frequently to give Mary a break and to walk with me as I tried to gain strength walking in circles with my walker on the driveway.

We were told that whenever we went anywhere, that I had to ride in the backseat, so that my torso and the LVAD would not be struck by an airbag in case of accident. As I gained strength, and we were able to get around, I became a terrible "backseat driver." I agreed that Mary was a fully capable driver, but I thought she constantly needed my verbal help. Eventually, she had enough. One day, she pulled to the side of the street, stopped the car, and looked in the rearview mirror. She said, "If you don't shut up and quit telling me how to drive, I am going to put you out and leave you right here!" I shut up.

Our most memorable moment with Mary driving and me riding in the back seat came a few days later. Mary wanted to drive to Greenville, Texas and check on Horace Graham, her elderly second cousin. This 75 mile trip appealed to me, so I assured her that I would be careful with my back seat driving tendencies. We had just traded for another used car and I was anxious to see how it drove on the highway.

We lingered in our visit with Horace, and it was getting late in the day when we finally headed west to Denton on busy U.S. highway 380. 380 is only two lanes for the early portion of the trip and has constant traffic–especially a lot of trucks. When we went through Farmersville, I could see from the back seat that the gas gauge needle had suddenly gone to empty. I spoke up urgently and told Mary I thought we needed gas. When she looked at the gauge, she was surprised. Just a minute before, when she checked the gauge it showed more than half full. What we did not know until this moment was that this vehicle had a problem with the gas gauge. We were absolutely on empty and just at this moment realized it.

"What should we do" Mary asked. I told her I thought we had better pull off at a side road we were approaching and turn around and go back into town to get gas. As she turned onto the side right road and turned around, we knew that it would be very difficult to get back on the busy highway going the opposite direction. As we sat waiting for traffic to give us a "window," we crafted a plan. I would watch for traffic one direction and she the other. When the "window of opportunity" came, she would "gun" the accelerator and move quickly into the traffic. The "window" came and Mary pressed the accelerator. Nothing happened. The car was completely out of gas. Traffic was whizzing by us just a couple of feet in front of our car!

Mary immediately put the car flashers on. In a few minutes, there was a car that pulled off and turned and pulled up behind us. A man came to the window to see if he could help. He explained that he had just been to Farmersville to see his parents and was on his way home to Plano. He was a nice man– about our age - and seemed trustworthy. He offered to drive

Mary back into Farmersville so she could buy a gas can and get gas to put in the car. Mary got in the car with the man and they drove away.

I didn't realize immediately the spectacle that I was: a very large man, sitting in the back seat of a car with the flashers on, just a couple of feet from the whizzing traffic. I was thankful to have an adequate supply of spare batteries for my LVAD. So I sat, the only noise in the car the *swish swish* sound from the LVAD vent. I noticed in a few minutes that an old van with two elderly ladies was slowing to turn off the highway to investigate what was going on. Soon they had pulled up and parked behind me. At this exact moment, the alarm sounded on my LVAD controller, indicating that the batteries needed changing. As I reached for the big black bag that contained my spare batteries, one of the ladies approached the car. It was a hot summer day, and Mary had left me with the windows down so that I would not get too hot. The little gray haired lady looked in my window at me. Only in later reflection did I realize that I surely looked to her like something from outer space. The car flashers were on, the controller on my belt was sounding an alarm, I had wires attached to my body, I had large black straps holding big batteries under my arms, and the noise from the LVAD was going *swish swish*. The lady stammered, "Do you need help, sir?" I told her that I just needed to change my batteries. The truth of my situation was beyond her ability to grasp. All she heard was the word "battery" and she thought I was in a desperate emergency. She quickly said, "Do we need to go into town and get you a 'bat-rey'?" I tried to calm her and explain that I was okay. I quickly changed the batteries and the alarm went off. Then I told her that my wife had gotten a ride into town with someone to get gas for our car. This kind little lady seemed so desperately worried about me. "Don't you need our help?" she wanted to know. I assured her that I would be okay. "We could stay with you," she said. Again I assured her that everything would be fine. She walked away slowly.

In about fifteen minutes, Mary returned with the man and a full can of gas. As he put the gas into the car for her, Mary leaned in the open window and asked me what the old van with the two ladies was doing parked behind me. Only at that moment did I realize these two ladies had ignored my assurances that I was okay, and had stayed *with me.* Soon we were on the road to the next town with the man following us closely until we stopped at a station and filled up with gas. When the tank was full, the man gave Mary a business card, just in case something further happened and we needed his help. As Mary pulled back into the traffic, headed to Denton, we began to reflect on the significance of the three strangers–who had been *with us* on this hot summer day. I recalled the afternoon when Matt Nelson had been *with me.* And I had recalled how others along the way, especially the Bernards, had traveled such a long way to be *with me.*

What emerged in my meditations as we drove down the road was that the literal truth of Psalm 23 had been lived in my life the past 8 months. The Psalmist had said, "…though I walk through the valley of the shadow of death, I will fear no evil, for Thou art *with me.*" In my situation, on the lonely day of desperation in Baylor Hospital eight months before, Matt Nelson had been *with me.* That was the day I entered the valley of the shadow of death, I now realized. Finally on this strategically important day of my journey to four hearts, three strangers had been *with me.* This was at the end of this journey through the valley of the shadow of death. God had been with me through this journey as he promised. I believed I would live, as I had seen God at my side in the persons of these precious people.

We made regular trips back to Baylor over the next few weeks. I was making good progress. We learned by trial and error to keep the batteries charged, to get the dressing changed, and to carry the right number of batteries and the manual pump with us.

Our family had a nice celebration on July Fourth. A few months before, I would not have imagined that I would be alive to sing the national anthem again.

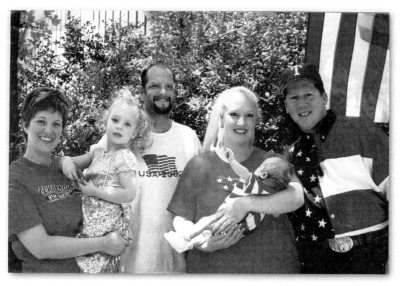

DLynn, Tatum, Dave, Rachel, A.J., and Clint on July 4, 2005.
Dave would not be with us to sing the national anthem the next year

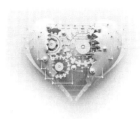

DRIVING

I realized that I was gaining strength when I began to want to drive. I had been told it would be a long wait. There were so many issues. How would I be able to handle the situation if I were driving alone and my LVAD quit? Dr. Kuiper told me that I would have to pass a "test" to be able to drive. By early August, I wanted to try the test to see if I could drive. Dr. Kuiper explained that I would have to come to Baylor and be admitted to the hospital to take the test. This was a really unusual kind of driving test. It had nothing to do with driving. It was all about how long I could make it if my LVAD went out. This was a dangerous thing to do and they wanted me in a hospital environment if something went wrong. After I was admitted and taken to a room, a nurse put an IV in with some fluid and medication of some kind, and then Dr. Kuiper came in. He explained that when we were ready, he would have me stand up and then he would turn off the LVAD. Then he would use the manual pump to pump six times a minute for twenty minutes. I had to be able to stand that long without blacking out and with almost no blood supply. We started and my head soon began to spin. I was determined and so, to keep myself going, I began to tell Dr. Kuiper all the funny jokes and stories that I could think of. Although I was very dizzy at the end, I made it. The point of the process is to prove if there is an accident while driving that I had sufficient strength to do without the LVAD and very minor manual pumping long enough to get out of harm's way. I still enjoy telling Dr. Kuiper jokes and funny stories.

Again, those months seemed like I was living in a cocoon, isolated from the world around me. On one of my first drives, we drove by Presbyterian Hospital, where we heard our friend, Jane Mann, had been hospitalized. Our families had, for many years, celebrated New Year's Eve with the Manns, the Landreths, and the Davises. Mary and Jane had been hospitalized together at old Flow Hospital in Denton almost thirty-six years before, having their respective children, David and Jim. I sat outside in the car while Mary tried to find out about Jane. She didn't see her and didn't get much information. In a couple of days we heard that Jane had died. This was such a shock to us. Jane had always seemed so healthy and then, after a brief illness, she was gone. Life continues to be a mystery ... how someone so precariously close to death can live and then someone so healthy dies without warning.

David visited with Rachel a lot that summer while she was on maternity leave. She remembers him bringing her food or coffee, but mostly encouragement for taking care of a new baby. A.J. would follow in Tatum's footsteps to Children's Corner when Rachel returned to work in September. That summer was difficult for Clint as his father, Al, had a lengthy series of illnesses and was hospitalized for several months. He had some diabetes complications and had endured an amputation. He died, and his funeral was on Friday, September 13. It was a tough loss for Clint and his family.

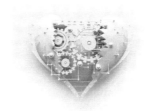

FRIDAY NIGHT

I had another memorable moment that night. I was now able to get around with a cane and my friend, Gene Conyers, came to get me to take me to the high school football game. Clint and I had season tickets beside Gene. As the game was about to kick off, Clint called me. Rachel had gone to her monthly Bunko group, and he asked what I thought about him bringing three-month-old A.J. to the football game. I told him to come on. I had the tickets and would enjoy holding A. J. In a little while, they were with us at the ballgame. It was good for Clint. Gene and I had dubbed him "the Nacho Kid" because of his nacho-eating prowess at baseball games. He was ready to go to the concession stand when they got to the stadium. I held A.J. It had only been three months since A.J. had welcomed me home by wetting on me. I enjoyed watching him look around, trying to figure out all the noise and excitement. It was a very emotional moment for me. Just five months before, I thought I would die. Now, in this familiar, enjoyable place, I asked God for a new desire of my heart. I became oblivious to the game. I asked God to allow me to live long enough to see A.J. as a high school football player on the field below while I watched from this same seat. By now, A.J. was fast asleep. It seemed to me that night that God said yes. Time will tell.

David was ever persevering. I found out from DLynn that while things were so bad with me back in the spring, Dave had a lot of challenges in Milwaukee at the Harley parts catalog shoot. She said when he got to the hotel at night, the sores on his feet and legs had leaked so much that he actually had blood-soaked socks. All through the summer, he was going to Lewisville to get treatment on his sores. They were not getting better. He was just persevering. He had been an encouragement to Rachel, and he always enjoyed Tatum. He was not working, so finances were a challenge. Jim Mann had asked him to video Jane's funeral for his family, and David did so.

In early October, he called me and told me that he was on the way over and bringing me a book he wanted me to read. He and Jim had had lunch and Jim had given him the book for doing the funeral video. The book, by Don Piper, was titled *90 Minutes in Heaven*. Dave was such an avid reader. He would start a book and read it in one sitting. I could tell that this book had impacted him in an unusual way. I read it right away and it had the same impact on me. It is the true story told by Pastor Don Piper, who had a head-on collision with an eighteen-wheeler in his little Ford Escort. He was mangled and pronounced dead, left with a tarp over him while EMTs attended to other injured. Only after ninety minutes had passed did another pastor, a bystander, discover that Don was alive. Yet during those ninety minutes, Don had been in heaven and recalled it vividly. Then he spent thirteen horrendous months in a contraption that kept him alive and evoked excruciating pain. I was challenged, as was Dave, not by the 25 percent of the book that talked about what heaven was like as much as the 75 percent of the book that described the hell on earth of living through the pain and suffering. The book so influenced me that I began to order them by the box and give them to people that I knew.

Our church had a fall 5K-run called the "Harvest Haul" on October 15. I determined to walk one mile with my cane. I did the mile-walk in thirty minutes, thanks to the encouragement of John Duncan and Verl Young, who walked along beside me.

I wanted to take our family to Beaver's Bend that fall, just to have a little time away. We had to make considerable preparation. Beaver's Bend is in southeastern Oklahoma, about a three-hour drive from home. Some of the cabins at Beaver's Bend are older, so first we had to call and be sure that our family cabin had three-pronged outlets for plugging the LVAD base unit into. Some did and some didn't. We were assured that they would work with us to be sure that our family had one that worked. We had to load all the equipment and dressing-change materials. Clint helped us load our things and all their baby things for A.J. David came and brought Tatum, but DLynn couldn't come because of her school teaching schedule. We enjoyed the wildlife and a hike along the running river. Dave brought his bicycle and enjoyed riding it through the leaves in the gleaming autumn sunlight. Tatum was curious about everything there. Mary and I enjoyed watching Tatum and holding A.J. Dave marinated some steaks, and grilled a wonderful meal for us. Clint got a blazing campfire going and we sat around the fire, singing songs and roasting marshmallows. Those two days are a wonderful memory of David full of joy.

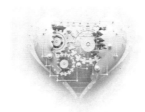

THANKSGIVING 2005

I wanted to help Dave see if he couldn't get some business locally since all the Harley things were so hard for him to do. He needed a location where he could have his equipment and a chance to hopefully do some personal photography, like weddings. It had just not been affordable for him to do, so in November, he and I looked at an old remodeled service station. He loved it. I decided to lease the space and offer to share it with him. I signed the lease, effective January 1, 2006. We were given permission to start moving some things in. I went to Hobby Lobby and got a collection of picture frames for him so he could frame some of his work and display it on the walls. He was very encouraged.

When Thanksgiving came, we all traveled to Floydada, Texas, to my sister Molly's, where we had shared many Thanksgivings. We had many things to be thankful for that year. I was living successfully with an LVAD. We had a new grandchild. David was encouraged about the new business thing that was going on. My brother-in-law, Jack Boggs, was in rare form as we watched football, played "42," and ate a bountiful meal. Our whole family enjoyed hearing him once again exclaim, "Man, this is really living!" He had just partially retired from the pastorate, and he and my sister, Jo, had bought a house and moved to Floydada. We marked the occasion by Dave taking an old-fashioned, black-and-white, group picture out on the driveway. He enjoyed getting everyone situated. He was the one who coined the phrase, "front row" for my siblings and me. He said that in all the old family group photos, the oldest generation was sitting in chairs on the front row with the following generations standing behind and the kids sitting or kneeling in front. So he arranged us that way and set up the tripod and the camera to take the picture. He pressed the button and got in the picture. It snapped in a few seconds. The picture became a treasured family heirloom.

David commemorated the photo as a celebration of the 75th anniversary of Joe and Opal Earp, who had married in 1930. He traced the outline of the picture, and on each silhouette, he printed the name of the person. Then he placed this "map" of all the people on the back of the photo. One of the frustrations that he had often seen was in various family members trying to figure out who all the people were in old family photos. He solved the problem for anyone who would look at this photo, generations later. Dave carefully made one of the photos for all of our family in the picture.

Back in Denton, we spent much of December preparing and moving into the building. We had often laughed about the "Governor" story, so I got a big frame and asked him if he would make a special picture of the "Governor" to display in the frame. We had a lot of fun planning this local shoot. The idea of the shoot was to make it seem as if the "Governor of Texas," in a big cowboy hat, was standing in front of the capital with his beloved "Queen" next to him, all decked out in her sequined evening attire, with long white gloves, and lots of lipstick and makeup. Mary was game for it and began to collect all of her props. Part of our planning was to figure out how to take the picture and hide all of the wires, straps, and batteries, so there was no indication that the "Governor" had an LVAD. David decided if he used the Denton County courthouse on the square as a background, it would look somewhat like the State Capitol Building in Austin. We met a few days before Christmas on the square. Mary and I were in our costumes. David had all his gear. We figured out that if I took the battery harness off and held the batteries in one hand behind Mary, any evidence of the LVAD would be shielded. We posed and David snapped away. It would be the last picture he took of us.

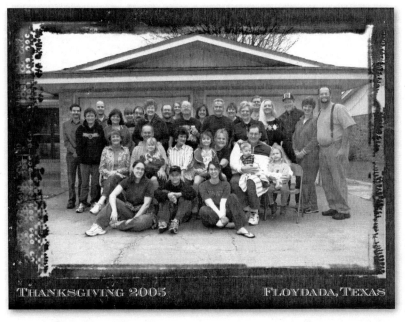

The "front row" – Wes, Jo, Molly, and James. This is the last
Thanksgiving we had Jack (middle, behind Jo) and David (far right) with us.

We enjoyed Christmas. Dave told us that between Christmas and New Year's, he was going to drive south and do some location scouting for the Harley spring shoot. When he got back he told me that they had decided to base their shoot in Round Rock. He had found several places that were ideal for the shoot. And he told me that he wanted to go and help with the shoot.

Mary noticed that when we were together on New Year's Day, he didn't act like he felt well.

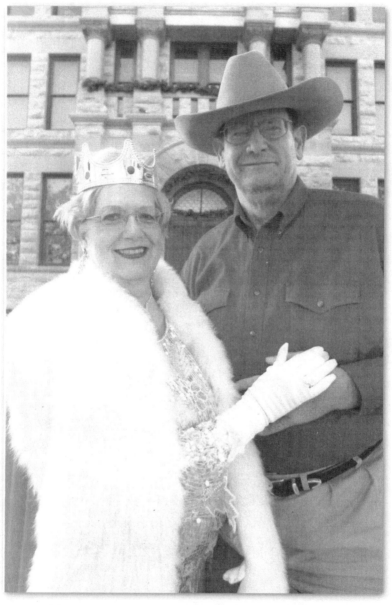

The Governor and the Queen – Dave's last photo of us

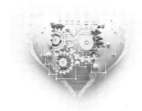

ROUND ROCK

Dave insisted on packing up and going the next day, January 2, 2006. He told me that when he got back in a few weeks, he would get the "Governor's" picture hung and settle into his new location.

Two days later, Mary talked to him on the phone and he wasn't feeling well. DLynn heard on Thursday that he was sick in the hotel room. Then on Friday she got a call from Trudy Bastman, the art director again on the shoot. David was at St. David's hospital in Round Rock. Trudy had called 911. DLynn immediately left for Round Rock, about 220 miles from Denton. We picked up Tatum.

DLynn called our house that night in a panic. The ER doctor had tried to do a spinal tap several times, without success. Finally, when he had success, spinal fluid had spewed all over the ER. Dave's life was in the balance once again. After the spinal fluid episode, the ER doctor decided that Dave had spinal meningitis. DLynn had already called her mother, who was on the way from Louisiana.

The next morning we loaded all our equipment and supplies and drove to Round Rock. Over the weekend, Dave rallied and was moved to a regular hospital room. As we were able to talk to him, we hoped this was just another of the Harley-shoot crises.

Maybe if we could get him well enough to get back to Denton, he would be okay.

We got a room in the Hilton hotel where the crew was staying. It was a short drive to the hospital. DLynn was using Dave's room at the same hotel. One of DLynn's challenges was that she had missed so much time due to past illnesses that she needed to be back in Denton to teach school the next week. Mary and I decided we could stay. We had all our clothes, equipment, and plenty of batteries. DLynn planned to come back on Friday, as it would be the beginning of the Martin Luther King holiday weekend.

Mary and I alternated staying with David. I would go early in the morning and then go back to the hotel where she did the dressing change on me. Then we packed plenty of batteries and headed back to the hospital. She would stay in the room with David and I would sit in the lobby. None of our cell phones worked inside the hospital, so I would go outside to make calls and check our messages.

On Tuesday the doctors took Dave off steroids. We realize now that was a big mistake. St. David's was a smaller hospital and the doctors and staff did not have a clear understanding of Dave's challenging history. We began to wish that we had him back at Baylor with the familiar doctors who knew his condition so well.

The staff tried really hard to deal with Dave's situation. His sores were so problematic. He needed the special support hose that we had only been able to find in Dallas, so a friend from Denton went to Dallas and got them and brought them to us. We were blessed by so many friends and family helping us in this new crisis.

My emotions ebbed and flowed. It was painful to see my son and his family in such a mess. Dave was good at his profession.

DLynn was a good teacher. They were great parents to Tatum. They were faithful in their personal lives and in their church. They had endured one terrible crisis after another. Yet they were plagued with medical bills and financial challenge. Their old van was not trustworthy for DLynn to be driving as far as Round Rock. Their peers were driving new cars and moving to bigger houses. They were healthy. I began to get a new case of "life is not fair." One of the ways I helped as I had the time to stand outside was to use my cell phone to call and try to settle some of the huge medical bills Dave and DLynn had hanging over them. I worked with the billing group at St. David's to work out a solution to the bill Dave would have there. In my thought-life, I seethed with anger.

Thursday, January 12, I saw an article in the Round Rock newspaper with Don Piper's picture on the front page. That very day he was in Round Rock at a book signing at the HEB super-market. I showed the article to Dave and we recalled the impact of the book in our lives, even as we were living in the same kind of suffering that Don Piper had lived through.

I sat in the lobby after lunch. David napped in his room, Mary at his side. I looked up to see Bob Billups and Mike Green from our church staff. They had driven all the way from Denton to be with us. Bob is a jovial guy, the senior associate pastor of our church. His way is to kid and joke about things. I am sure he was not prepared for the hour-long angry explosion that I unloaded on him. Where was God? He was not fair! Go back to Denton and tell that preacher of ours that tithing doesn't work! Why did everyone else have good health and prosperity? On and on I went. I cannot remember ever in my life unloading on anyone the way I did that day. Bob just looked at me kindly and listened. Finally I was done. I felt better. He took my hand and prayed with me. He and Mike made a quick trip upstairs to

Dave's room and shared a word with Mary. Then they headed back to Denton.

David's feet and legs were on fire that evening. Mary and I sat on either side of him at the foot of the bed, using ice and cool washcloths to try to give him some relief. We lingered late and went to the hotel and went to bed.

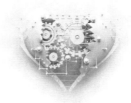

STROKES AND PARALYSIS

The next morning was a cool sunny Friday, January 13th. It was the beginning of the Martin Luther King holiday weekend. I left Mary resting and drove to the hospital early. David was not awake. I just sat, waiting for him to wake up. The nursing shift changed and we were alone for a long time. He seemed to rouse, but couldn't quite seem to wake up. Time passed. The nurse for the day breezed in and greeted me and wrote a couple of things on the chart. I began to worry about Dave. He still was drowsy and not alert. I pressed the nurse's call-button and waited for a while. I pressed it again. The nurse returned and I explained my concern. She looked more closely at David, and then called the doctor.

As the doctor shined his light into Dave's glazed eyes, he softly told me that he believed that David had had a stroke over-night. In fact, David had had five strokes since the night before. It would take long into the afternoon with multiple tests and an MRI to confirm that. The ICU was full and a special place was made for Dave in the ER where he lay, totally unconscious, on a ventilator.

We had called DLynn as soon as we realized what was hap-pening. By 4 p.m. a chaplain was with the three of us at Dave's bedside. It seemed that he might die any minute. In that moment, we prepared that his death was imminent. Several of the staff came by, a counselor and another chaplain among them, and gave us their business cards. They said to call them if "something happened" over the weekend. Since it was a holiday weekend, many of them would not be around. We understood what they meant.

Somehow as the hours passed, David pulled through. Mary and I were exhausted and emotionally drained, and we went to the hotel to get some sleep. DLynn stayed at David's side. About 2 a.m. we were awakened by a very loud and unfamiliar noise. It was the LVAD base unit that I was attached to. We did not know what the problem was, and we could not get the noise to quit. It was loud enough that we were afraid other people in the hotel would be disturbed. Even when we turned the unit off, the noise continued! Finally, I unplugged the unit, and the noise quit. We tried turning the machine off and on and doing various things. Our conclusion was that the LVAD base unit had failed. While we had quite a few charged batteries, we realized that we did not have the emergency twenty-four-hour battery pack with us. We had never needed it, so with the stress of the situation, we had left home without it!

We dressed and went to the hospital. Mary sat with David, and I got on the phone to try to figure out what to do about the LVAD power base unit. Since the cell phone did not work in the hospital, I stood outside in the dark and called the emergency number at Baylor Medical in Dallas and got Susan on the line. It was about 3 a.m. and I had calculated that I had enough battery capacity to last until about 7 p.m.

This happened to be Susan's first experience at being on-call for the heart failure clinic on a holiday weekend. Susan explained that the backup LVAD base unit had been pressed into service the night before at Baylor and so was unavailable. We discussed various things to try, all of which I had already tried. She speculated that they would have to order another LVAD base unit from the manufacturer after the holiday. I quickly got into panic mode, yelling at her over the phone that I only had enough battery capacity to last until 7 p.m. and couldn't wait until next week for a replacement! She seemed to shift into another gear mentally and told me she would see what she could do and would call me back. We talked several times in those early morning hours.

I began to try to think of all the other things that I could do. I thought about trying hospitals in Austin or San Antonio, closer to where we were, but I found out there were no LVAD base units in either place. I remembered that my brother, Wes, and his wife, who also live in Denton, were leaving Denton at 5 a.m. to drive down and spend the day with us. I was able to reach them on their cell phone. They were already halfway to Fort Worth. I quickly explained the emergency and asked them to turn around and go back to our house and get the twenty-four-hour emergency backup pack, which would buy us another twenty-four hours. By 10 a.m., Susan reported that a replacement LVAD base unit was being flown in from the manufacturer in California, to arrive in Dallas later in the day. We felt a little more at ease, knowing that the twenty-four-hour emergency pack was on the way.

Through the morning, as the word spread about David, we began to have various family and friends arrive to be with us. I stood outside, anxiously waiting for my brother. At about 11 a.m., my brother arrived. For the first time ever, I opened the top of the emergency backup pack to hook it up. The compartment at the top was empty, and I could not find a cable to connect it. Only later did we remember that the special cable was stored away at home with some other things and not in the compartment on the top of the unit. I had been told about that when I first came home, but now it was nine months later and I had no memory of being told that. So we had the emergency pack, but no cable to hook it up. This is not a cable that you get a replacement for at the hardware store. So our only option was the replacement LVAD base unit that was on a flight on its way to Dallas, 200 miles away!

Mark Harmer of the Harley crew joked that they could line the crew up and take turns pumping the manual pump! But God's mercy and grace came into play again as we remembered that our friends, John and Kay Duncan from Denton, were planning to come to see us later in the day. So I called and asked them to go to Baylor Hospital on the way and Susan arranged to meet them there. They all waited together in the heart unit at Baylor until the LVAD base unit arrived about 3 p.m. By 6:30 p.m., they were in Round Rock with the replacement unit and some spare batteries. At that point, my last battery had alarmed!

Dave's condition was stable, but unchanged. Our thought and desire was about how and when we could get him to Baylor in Dallas where they were more familiar with his history. DLynn's sister had come from Louisiana to be with her. We had a large group surrounding us in the chapel of the hospital. We prayed for a way to get Dave back to Dallas.

By Sunday morning, a place had opened for Dave in ICU. DLynn spent the day at David's side. He seemed a little better. He was able to interact and gave signs of slight improvement. He was at least partially paralyzed. His mouth and his right side had been affected by the strokes.

The Harley crew sensed our need for a break, so they encouraged Mary and me to drive out to their shoot in front of an old barbecue restaurant a few miles away. Our friend Tom Thornton from Austin called and wanted to see us, so we gave him directions to the shoot location. Tom joined us as we watched Madison Ford and his assistants get the motorcycle lighted and then click away when the sun got close to sundown.

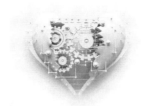

BACK TO BAYLOR

By late Monday morning, I had made all the insurance calls and contacts that were necessary for getting David back to Baylor. The transportation arrangements were with a local ambulance service. The staff at St. David's had done their best, but they were ready to release David to somewhere more familiar with him. Mary and I had been in Round Rock for ten days and we were ready to leave. Several of Dave's friends on the shoot helped us gather our equipment and get loaded up at the hotel. The ambulance service came to the hospital about 2 p.m. and began the preparation process to take Dave to Dallas. They were not familiar with Dallas, so I offered to lead them in a caravan. I was concerned about DLynn in Dave's old van, so she followed me, with the ambulance behind her. It was just turning dark as our caravan pulled onto the Baylor campus.

Dave stayed in the stroke ICU unit for a week. Dr. LaBeche conducted all the tests to evaluate the strokes and pinpoint where they had occurred and what the damage had been. She said that he had actually had seven strokes. The supposition was that if Dave's only problem had been spinal meningitis, taking him off steroids after the fourth day would have been okay. However, with all his other medical issues and transplant background, that likely contributed to the strokes. Dave was paralyzed totally on the right side. Because the right side of his mouth was paralyzed, his speech was slurred. By the end of the week, plans were made to move Dave across the street to .Baylor Institute for Rehabilitation (BIR).

Dave's BIR experience was a mixture of the good, the bad, and the ugly. He would have every kind of therapy to bring his damaged and paralyzed body to functionality. He tried with great effort, but it never happened.

Our church family and friends had rallied around us again. With their generosity, and the help of a local car dealer, we were able to get a good used van that would be reliable for DLynn to drive back and forth to Dallas. We settled into a routine as she taught school during the week, coming for the group therapy meetings that were held on Mondays. Mary and I traded out days being with Dave, and Rachel came when she could now that we were in the area.

Tatum's fourth birthday in February was a much-needed distraction for all of us. The party was at the Denton recreation center and there was a jump house and a "Thomas the Train" theme. Tatum had a small Thomas the Train engine, but it needed a battery that was not readily available. I found a battery store in Lewisville that had a battery that would work, bought it, and started to leave the store. The owner of the store was intrigued by my LVAD and batteries and began to ask lots of questions. I showed him the batteries. He was curious to see if he might have a battery in the store that would work with the LVAD. He found a battery that looked similar. I replaced one of my batteries with it and it worked! Then he showed me that he had a charger that could be plugged into the cigarette lighter in the car. An LVAD battery could be recharged in the car in two hours in an emergency. I bought one of these chargers to give us some additional backup in case we had any further problems. Before I left, he gave me his card and assured me that I could call him anytime of the day or night if I had an emergency and he would help me.

On the day of the party, Thomas the Train worked with his new battery. Mary helped me get myself together as "Sir Top-pam Hat" with batteries!

We had a great time. My brother Wes went to get David from BIR and he sat at the party in his wheelchair, enjoying being away from BIR. The party gave lots of people a chance to greet him for the first time since he had left Denton on January 2. Dave enjoyed more the little party that DLynn planned on Tatum's real birthday in the conference room at BIR. There was just our close family there: DLynn, Tatum, Rachel, Clint, Mary, and me. The joy for Dave was in getting some great time individually with Tatum. He loved calling her "Baby."

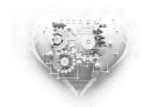

JACK LEAVES THE FRONT ROW

I answered the phone on Sunday evening, February 26, to the shocking news that my great friend and "really living" brother-in-law, Jack Boggs, had died. He had preached in church that morning and died that night. Mary and I loaded up our equipment and supplies once again and headed to Floydada to comfort our sister, Jo, and her family. We arrived with our suburban having a problem so we had to take it directly to the dealer in Floydada for repair.

The sanctuary at First Baptist Church in Floydada was almost full on the day of the funeral service, as pastor friends and congregants from over the years came to honor and remember this much beloved pastor. My sister told me that there were dozens of ministers who would love to conduct the funeral, but she knew that Jack would want me to because of our decades of sharing the most intimate spiritual thoughts. So I conducted the funeral. In such a setting, I had to carefully prepare myself not just spiritually but emotionally, mentally, and physically so my speaking was clear and projected above the noise of the LVAD "swish swish." The congregation hardly noticed the noise. We rejoiced at a great life that had been lived and grieved at the great loss for those left behind. We shared a brief lunch with family afterwards.

Then we got our repaired suburban, loaded our equipment and headed for BIR in Dallas. I was in a hurry to get there and was driving too fast. A young highway patrolman stopped us, looked at my license, and my batteries, and asked where I was going in such a hurry. I told him. He handed me my license and said to get on down the way, but be careful.

There began to be indications from the BIR staff that Dave had reached the limit of what they might do for him. They were good at rehabbing people who had been injured or had just had a stroke. They did not seem to know how to treat him medically with all his sores and medical history. I could tell they wanted to find a way to move David out of their care.

These were hard, grueling days. Other LVAD patients were focused on staying alive. I was focused on watching helplessly as every shred of life unraveled for David. Some people mentioned to me that I was like Job in the Bible. I didn't relish such thought and pity by others. No one seemed to know what to say. Long gone were the days when others reassured that "it will get better soon." Even as I walked down the hall at church, some people who saw me a long way off would turn and go the other way, just to not have to encounter me. It seemed to me as if I were a lightening rod, and that people feared getting too close to me, afraid they would be struck by lightening also.

The good and the bad happened in March. Mary saw a note one Friday afternoon at the bookstore in Denton that Don Piper, the author of the *90 Minutes in Heaven* book would be speaking at seven the next evening at a church in Forestburg, Texas, almost an hour northwest of Denton. We decided that we wanted to go. The next morning I drove to BIR to be with Dave and told him that we were planning to go hear Don Piper speak that night. Immediately Dave pleaded with me that he wanted to go. That he might want to go had not even occurred to me.

Yet he had been the one who had gotten me onto the book and ordering them by the box. My initial response was, "It's not possible." Dave pleaded, "Come on Dad, please try." Of course I would try to help him do something that he really wanted to do. I found the charge nurse and explained the request. This was on the weekend so there was no therapy scheduled. The charge nurse was an older man, very laid back, who had openness to this. He explained that Dave was inpatient and that he absolutely had to be in his bed at midnight for insurance purposes. Otherwise, as far as he was concerned, Dave could go and he would help me load him and his wheelchair into my vehicle downstairs. I shared with Dave the midnight requirement and that getting back in time would be tight, considering how far away Forestburg was. He was determined to go.

By seven p.m. five of us, Dave, DLynn, Tatum, Mary and I, were seated near the front of the church, waiting to hear Don Piper speak. David was in his wheelchair in the aisle at the end of the pew where the rest of us were seated. The church was packed. The previous weekends Don had been in Sweden, Detroit, and Chicago. Now he was in a little church in Forestburg, Texas. And Dave was there. Amazing! About halfway into Don's message, Dave leaned over and whispered something to DLynn. Don Piper was in a suit and tie and looked perfectly healthy except for a slight limp. He spoke powerfully and effectively from his heart. People lined up afterwards to buy a book and get his autograph. Dave made it clear to me that he wanted to stay and visit with Don and his wife. I told him we would try but we had to be back to BIR by midnight! While we waited, Mary chased Tatum around. She was having a great time. Dave and DLynn enjoyed visiting in this new context. I occupied our place at the end of the line. And then the moment Dave wanted came. We all huddled around Don and his wife and shared some of our story. We already knew a lot of their story from the book. Don saw that Dave was paralyzed and immediately reached his right hand straight out to shake Dave's hand. I watched as Dave struggled with all his might to lift his right hand to take Don's. He got it partially lifted and Don reached and grabbed it and shook it. Dave asked Don if he still had pain. "All the time," Don replied. "I am never without it."

Then DLynn laughed and asked Don if he had seen Dave whispering to her. Yes, he had. DLynn told Don, "he whispered, 'I wonder what he looks like naked.'" We all laughed, knowing that Don had been so severely injured that his body was a mess with major reconstructions throughout his body. Don smiled and said, "Dave, you don't need to see me naked. Just look at this." Don took off his jacket and rolled up his left shirt-sleeve. He held his "naked" left arm high in the air. It was a grotesque layering of sinew and grafting. It was terrible to look at, to the point that I wanted to turn away and not look. Don Piper had struck a chord with Dave. He took comfort in knowing the pain that Don Piper lived with. Don wrote Dave a note: "See you at the gate! Don Piper." We all prayed fervently together in a little huddle. No one else was around. This was the good. I hurried everyone to the car and dropped the girls off in Denton. When I got Dave to BIR, it was a quarter of midnight. I called the nurse who came down and helped me get Dave in his wheelchair and to the second floor. We had made it with minutes to spare.

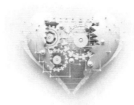

HANGING ON TO LIFE

We began to see that we might be bringing David home in a wheelchair. A group of friends began to work to modify Dave and DLynn's home to make it wheelchair friendly. I checked out the cost and feasibility of having the van modified for wheelchair accessibility. The money to pay for a new life at home for a totally disabled person was a big challenge. Rachel visited with Dave and decided she would do a fundraiser by planning to run the White Rock Marathon in December. She would ask people to donate so much a mile for Dave's benefit.

The old prankster Dave came to life in one of Rachel's visits. He had always been her nemesis, even from when the time he was only a year and a half old when she was born. As she softly stepped into his room at BIR to check on him, he began to convulse, roll his eyes, and act like a crazy person. She panicked and started to run from the room to call the nurses. Dave started laughing. He had gotten his sister one more time!

Two times in March we had Dave in Denton in his wheelchair. These were the bad. One was for my sixtieth birthday party, which Mary and Rachel planned. The party itself was a joyful time of celebration. Many friends and family came to celebrate the extended life that I had with the LVAD. It again gave many people the opportunity to see Dave in his wheelchair. Although he enjoyed seeing so many people that he had not seen in a long time, he clearly had mixed feelings with them seeing him in the condition he was in. He ached for time with DLynn and was so sad to have to go back to BIR without that.

We tried again two days later. Some of our family was still together as we celebrated Rachel's thirty-fifth birthday. My sister, Jo, was with us and late in the day we started out to drive Dave back to BIR in her van. Torrential rains blocked the freeway and we moved to an alternate route down Harry Hines Boulevard to downtown. The rain was so bad we could hardly drive. And then something happened to my sister's van. We found ourselves parked in a parking lot at the side of Harry Hines, by now in the dark, in the pouring rain. My sister was still in grief, only a month after Jack's death. Dave was totally exhausted, really ready to get back to BIR. Thankfully I had plenty of batteries; my LVAD filled the silence with its swishing sound. I was thinking about what we were going to do. What a threesome we were, all of us were living through misery and suffering.

I decided to call my friend Gene Conyers to see if he was willing to come rescue us. I knew he had a vehicle and the driving skill that could navigate the high waters. Gene agreed to help, and about an hour later he pulled into the parking lot. We did our best to keep Dave from getting soaked in the transfer from Jo's van. By the time we got Dave to BIR, it was late on this Sunday night. He was soaked and exhausted. After we got him to his room on the second floor, he fell onto the bed and closed his eyes. He didn't even rouse to see us leave. Over the next couple of days the rain subsided, Jo's van got fixed, and she headed back to Floydada.

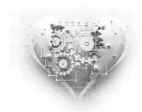

FACING REALITY

Mary and I had been invited to a conference in Las Vegas and thought being away a few days might be good. But it was a draining, not encouraging time. It was the first time we tried to take the LVAD base unit and all the equipment and supplies on a flight. We used the rolling walker that had belonged to Pop. The airport exhausted us, and it was late at night when we arrived at the hotel. We had already missed a nice dinner. The whole event was a disaster for us, trying to accommodate and use the equipment while "normal" people tried to help. A couple of days later, Mary and I sat alone in the hotel coffee shop and wept as we thought about David's precarious situation. Unbeknownst to us, while we were gone, at about the time we were weeping, Dave and DLynn were talking about his funeral plans.

The ugly began a few weeks later and lasted for six weeks. Dave's sores and medical issues got so bad at BIR that, in an emergency, he had to be brought to the ICU on the fourth floor of Collins, where he had had all his cancer treatment. This emergency brought about one of my most challenging battery experiences. As Mary and I worried in the fourth floor waiting room, many hours passed. I exhausted all the battery capacity that I had. I did not want to leave and go to Denton. Mary made some calls to see if there was an LVAD base unit available somewhere at Baylor so I could hook up and get my batteries charged. Finally, she discovered there was a unit in the ICU in Roberts that was not being used. A wheelchair was dispatched to Collins to get me and take me to the ICU in Roberts. The nurse who hooked me up that night and helped me get my batteries charged was Wendy Peavy, now my transplant coordinator almost four years later

Dave's condition was so fragile that even the best cancer nurses on the fourth floor were challenged. Dave's veins were impossible to get an IV in. A PICC line had to be inserted. Only with great skill and perseverance over a two-hour period was Dr. Capeheart finally able to get the line into Dave's groin. His photographer friend, Mark Harmer, had come to Dallas to see him and watched horrified at this episode. Dave was moved to ICU. The next night a group of young men from Dave's Sunday school class in Denton came to pray with him. Some of them were helping with the effort to modify Dave and DLynn's home to accommodate Dave's wheelchair. Dave rallied the next day. Insurance was always a factor and as soon as his medical condition seemed stable, he had to leave the ICU. I rolled him back through the tunnel under Gaston Avenue, to BIR.

Later this PICC line came out on a "field trip" that Dave and DLynn were taking as part of the rehab, trying to prepare for life away from BIR. This would prove to be the source of his worst infection. I was in the midst of a frustrating battle between the insurance company and the staff at BIR as to whether he was going to be forced to leave. Each side gave the view that it was "not them, but the other side" that was forcing Dave's removal from BIR. He was not able to go home. One extension was granted, but I was told on Monday, May 8, that we had until Friday, May 12, to find somewhere for Dave. A nursing home was the only option. I called all of the places that were on Dave's insurance. One in Plano agreed to look at all his records, as did one in Euless. On Tuesday, DLynn and I drove to Euless to see the one there. They initially agreed to take Dave. On Tuesday evening, I returned to Denton and went to the Denton Nursing Home and Rehabilitation Center. The people there were kind to stay late and visit with me and look at Dave's records, which I had with me. The medical director there just shook his head and told me directly that Dave's condition was so bad and complicated that he did not believe any nursing home would agree to take Dave.

The next morning, Mary's Aunt Hazel in Wellington was near death, so Mary decided she needed to make an overnight trip there to have a last visit. I drove to Dallas to continue the quest of finding a place for Dave. By noon, the nursing home in Euless had called and said after carefully reviewing Dave's records they would not be able to take him. Late in the afternoon, the nursing home in Plano that had seemed promising had called and said that they could not take Dave, either.

I was amazed that somehow DLynn had held up teaching school, coordinating the house remodeling for the wheelchair, and taking care of Tatum. In addition, she was faced with making the most gut-wrenching decisions about Dave. I called her and shared the bad news about all the nursing home options. We agreed our options had been exhausted. I wondered if on Friday, Dave would just be put in his wheelchair and wheeled to the curb. I offered to stay with Dave that evening and tell him.

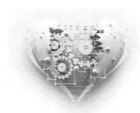

JESUS MAY COME TOMORROW

That night Dave and I had an amazing moment. I told him that none of the nursing homes were willing to take him and that come Friday, we did not know what would happen. He said, "Dad, don't worry. Jesus may come tomorrow!" He and I cried together and then prayed. I went home because my batteries were almost totally drained.

I went back to BIR early the next morning. I just took a few backup batteries, planning to be back in Denton by noon. I expected Mary back from Wellington because she had planned to pick up some things for Clint's thirty-seventh birthday party that night. The plan was that as soon as DLynn's last class was over, she would come to BIR and Mary and I would stay in Denton with Tatum to participate in Clint's party. Our family constantly juggled the issues of life, trying to live with some normalcy. The idea of a "new normal" meant that a birthday needed to be celebrated, even in the midst of difficulty.

There was a sign on David's door that morning saying that he was not to be disturbed, so I waited outside the door. I could hear activity in the room. Fifteen minutes passed, and I wondered what was going on. The nurse emerged and said that she had not been able to get a blood pressure reading on Dave since when she came on at seven.

The rest of the day was like living in slow motion. Nothing was being done. Had the doctor been called? Yes, he had. What would be done? Wait to hear from the doctor. Dave was unconscious with no blood pressure, but no one was doing anything. To figure out what to do, he would need a new PICC line. This meant a trip through the tunnel and then a two-hour wait to get the line. Multiple tries without success and still no line and still no blood pressure ... Back through the tunnel and to his room at BIR. I panicked and screamed, "Call the doctors in the cancer center!" They would know what to do. By 3 p.m. I was out of batteries. Finally I was told the cancer doctors would be called. Dave still lay unconscious, without a blood pressure. I now know that Dave was dying with a severe sepsis infection. As I went by the nurses' station, my batteries on amber alarm, I looked across at the BIR doctor. He did not want to look at me. I yelled at him that he needed to do something!

As I hurried to Denton, I updated DLynn on my cell phone as she was leaving Denton headed for Dallas. By 6 p.m. she had had one of the cancer doctor's walk over to BIR and take Dave back under the tunnel to the familiar fourth floor Collins ICU. A crisis doctor was on the way to his room. I got to Denton and got a fresh supply of batteries. Mary and I picked Tatum up, and took the items she had for the Clint's party by. We took a brief moment to wish Clint a happy birthday. Then we hurried to Dallas. About 7 p.m. we had arrived, and Mary went into Dave's room briefly. Then I went into Dave's room, and she occupied Tatum by looking at the fish in the aquarium in the familiar waiting room. Suddenly Dave's room exploded with alarms and all the nurses and staff started screaming, "Code purple! Code purple!" They rushed DLynn and me from the room. Dave was in cardiac arrest.

Dave was resuscitated after a long effort by the crisis doctor and staff. For the next two weeks, he would be on a ventilator. Only DLynn had any real connection with him during that period of time. Many family and friends came to visit. The fourth floor waiting room was once again a familiar place for our family. One of Dave's friends, his old roomy, Jeff Covieo, came from Michigan to visit. His other old roommate, Virgil Adams, and his family now lived near Baylor, and Virgil came to see Dave. DLynn, Tatum, Mary, and I spent the rest of May in an apartment at Twice Blessed House, where we had stayed many times before. So many school people called the administration to offer their "personal days" so that DLynn could be with Dave that the school district told DLynn to take the balance of the school year off.

There were two more gut-wrenching issues. Two weeks later, a decision had to be made to take Dave off the ventilator. Mary and I sat with DLynn in the ICU waiting room. She said, "The most challenging decision that most of my friends are making today is what color of new shoes to buy, and I have to decide to have the ventilator removed from my husband, knowing that he will die." We understood and agreed with the decision. The other was the task of telling her four-year-old daughter, Tatum, that her father was going to die. Shirley Jones, the preschool minister at our church came and brought a pamphlet about how to talk to a preschooler about death. She counseled with DLynn about what to say.

My soul was grieved to the core when Tatum cried that she wanted a daddy and if her daddy died, she wanted a new one. I continued an emotional battle with God. I pleaded with Him to allow David to live, so he could be a daddy to Tatum, and to take me. My life was marginal anyway. I had an LVAD "bridge to nowhere." Why couldn't He let Dave live, and take me? I had been prepared to die just a year before.

As I was thinking these thoughts, I was saddened to hear that Rachel Bernard, the only daughter and youngest child of Jacob and Claudette Bernard, had died. I grieved for them. I remembered how they had come close, all the way from Haiti, and prayed for me and cared for me just a year before. Mary and I would not be able to go and be a part of the funeral service or draw close to Jacob and Claudette as they had drawn close to us. We had not been able to travel to Haiti in the past few years. We could only pray for God's grace for them. We were with them in spirit if not in person.

I thought when they pulled the ventilator from Dave that he would die right away. It certainly seemed so. The familiar doctors and nurses all gathered in his room and cried and hugged all of our family as the vent was pulled. But Dave continued to hang on. His body was a shell of the big healthy one that I struggled to remember. Sunday, May 28, was DLynn's thirty-third birthday. Our family–Clint, Rachel, A.J., Mary and I–took DLynn and Tatum to the Dallas Arboretum just a couple of miles east of the Baylor campus, right on White Rock Lake. We ate lunch and strolled, watching the birds and looking at the flowers. This spot was one of DLynn and Dave's favorites.

We passed the time with intimate dialogue. Tatum watched videos at the apartment or the fish in the aquarium in the fourth floor Collins waiting room. Mary kept our laundry done, and sat in Dave's room in ICU, holding his hand, and whispering to him. DLynn read her Bible and sat up on the bed with Dave. I sat at the nurses' table outside Dave's room, typing on my laptop. I was working on his eulogy. Dr. Bryan Berryman, the doctor of the group who was "on" in May, stopped by often. He stood, quietly weeping, at my side the morning I was working on the eulogy.

On Monday night, as I sat with DLynn at the dining table of the apartment, she remarked, "You know, Grampsie, our family is living in God's favor." We discussed the biblical idea of "favor," especially from the book of Daniel, which she was studying.

On Tuesday, insurance issues forced us to begin exploring having Dave's care being taken over by hospice. It had been four days since Dave had been removed from the ventilator. He lingered, although his breathing was becoming very labored. On Tuesday night, a hospice representative came to the apartment to collect the information to start the process. When she left, DLynn and Mary went back to be with Dave, while I stayed in the apartment to get Tatum to bed.

Mary and DLynn had just come back to the apartment to get some sleep just after midnight. As they came in, Mary said to me that she wished she hadn't come back. She had told Dave when she left, "David, the angels are coming to get you." She hoped he understood. She didn't see how Dave was still living. Then a call came. Dave was in the process of dying, and so she and DLynn rushed back to the hospital. Tatum was asleep, so I waited at the apartment until our friends John and Kay Duncan came to stay with Tatum. I rushed to ICU, but Dave had already died in those early morning hours of May 31, 2006, even before the girls got back there. Rachel drove quickly from Denton to sit with us. We sat quietly staring at his lifeless body. I believed that he was alive, in heaven. However, the darkness of the night and the quiet sadness of the hours we sat there made the truth of eternity hard to grasp. I came to a new understanding of the words "hope" and "faith."

We returned to the apartment about 4 a.m. We slept briefly, and then DLynn got Tatum up and took her to Denton. Rachel, Mary, and I tarried. We had a lot to do. We made phone calls. Mary called Dr. Jeff and spoke with his wife Tami and told her that Dave had died.

The apartment had to be cleared. Rachel helped, and some family friends, Linda Davis, Lucy Wood, and Peggy Longworth, came and washed the sheets and cleaned the apartment. They packed DLynn and Tatum's things to take back to Denton. Mary and I sorted through the things in the refrigerator and packed items in an ice chest for Rachel to take back. We had all of our LVAD equipment–multiple bags of batteries, the base unit, and the dressing-change supplies that had to be sorted through and packed in our van, which was parked a long walk from the apartment. This difficult work was done quietly and efficiently. It marked one more time of a great number of times that we had close family and close friends at our side, helping get the menial necessary things done. What we would have done without the love and help of so many, I cannot fathom. When everything was loaded, and the apartment clean, the ladies left to come back to Denton. Mary and I returned the apartment keys and then decided that we needed to make a stop at Carr P. Collins Hospital.

We went to the clinic area on fifth floor of Collins. We paused in the waiting room, looking with fondness at Dave's pictures that he had made in Alaska, now hanging on the waiting room walls. We expressed our gratitude to everyone we saw for the care they had given Dave. We saw Freeman, "Dr. P" and his current nurse, Laura, and Ron, a most caring nurse. We took the elevator down to the fourth floor and saw some of the regular nurses and other staff. We went into ICU into the clean and dark room where Dave had died just a few hours before. We said "good-bye" to the room that now held so many of our family memories. We walked through the waiting room, pausing in front of the aquarium where we had sat so many times with each other and with Tatum. We saw Phyllis and others on this floor.

We left and went to Denton. Rachel was already back and hard at work getting the obituary ready for the newspapers.

The next days of our life are a blur. We constantly had people at our house, bringing food and sharing their love. The phone rang and rang. Relatives and friends descended on Denton to be with us. Though we were exhausted and bitterly grieved the love and kindness of our many family and friends and our church family helped.

Another "new normal" experience came on Friday night as our family gathered to celebrate A.J.'s first birthday.

The funeral home visitation was on Saturday, June 3. Derv Hudgins, the funeral director, suggested that there would be such a crowd at the visitation that we scheduled two different times, one at 2 p.m. and one at 5 p.m. Some friends brought sandwiches and refreshments for us so we could rest between times at the funeral home. Dave's photographer friends came and set up a memorial on an easel by Dave's casket. The abundance of flowers scented the large room and waiting area with a deep floral fragrance. The beauty of the flowers contrasted sharply with the severity of the loss.

Dave's funeral service was at our church on Sunday afternoon, June 4. The church was packed. We were surrounded with people, and held close in the loving arms of the Heavenly Father. As our family came up the aisle on the way out, we looked into the faces of so many who had stood with us for so long. I spied Willie Lafitte, all dressed in white, and remembered the morning just one year before when he came to my room and literally made me walk. I was now walking out of my son's funeral service. Willie, just a few days before, had come to Dave's ICU room to see if he could help with any kind of physical therapy for Dave. There were many others in the service that day. Willie's being there was a symbol of the care we felt from so many.

On the morning of June 5, our family had a private graveside service at Roselawn cemetery before Dave's burial. We sang "I'll Fly Away." We lingered at Roselawn as the morning sun softly glistened through the shade of the trees overhead. I marvel that it only takes half an hour to bury a life that took thirty six years to live. Since that morning Mary and I have returned many times to sit on a bench beside Dave's grave. It is a quiet place of solitude. We have since had chimes hung from a tree above the bench. The chimes are in "D major"—a fitting remembrance of our son.

Many of Dave's photographer friends from Michigan attended the private graveside service, and afterwards we went to the building where Dave's equipment still sat, never unpacked from the intended move-in. The friends helped DLynn sort through all of Dave's camera equipment to know what she might want to keep and what to sell.

Mary and I returned to our home and the people who collected there to deal with a new issue—the wooden floor in the kitchen buckled due to an ice chest leaking on it. Thankfully, by the end of the week our friend Don Barber had fixed it.

Our family brought food to the city park on June 13th and sat with DLynn to commemorate with her what would have been her eighth wedding anniversary. The next night we wore shirts that said "The Really Living Earps–remembering Dave and Jack" to the Texas Rangers baseball game. The Rangers recognized our group as the "Really Living Earps" on their outfield scoreboard.

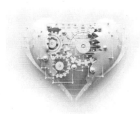

SUBMERGED IN GRIEF

I was not "really living" on the inside. I had put on lots of weight during the five month battle that was finished. It is a raw and bitter thing to lose a son. Mary and I were both on anti-depressants. We went through the motions day after day. We had to come to grips with the issue of what would happen to me. We were now into the second year with the LVAD and knew that it would wear out sometime. I had no thoughts of a heart transplant. That was an impossible issue for me. I would have to lose eighty pounds, and even then with all the matching issues of blood types and body sizes, the chances were slim. Here I was, living in depression with a mechanical pump pumping my blood. My only son was dead. I was hardly making it to the next day, much less finding the energy and will to lose weight. One of the people on the transplant team at Baylor suggested that I have a visit with Dr. Dee Rollins at Baylor Grapevine.

On Monday, June 26, 2006, Mary and I drove to Grapevine to visit with Dee Rollins. She appeared shocked as she saw us and our condition and heard our story. Her specialty is nutrition. She could be regularly seen on one of the network newscasts with her professional views on nutrition and eating disorders. She spent considerable time with us, just listening to our story. She expressed that she could hardly imagine how we were even there in our condition. She had never helped anyone who had been on an LVAD. I heard the unexpected from her that day. I had no expectation that there would be any value in this appointment. I saw myself as doing this to please my wife, a "going through the motions" kind of thing that held no hope at all. What I heard from her, like the still, small voice of God, gave me hope. She asked me if I thought I could live on 2,000 calories a day. I told her that I thought I could. And she gave me a sheet of paper and asked if I could keep a diary of all the calories I ate. I told her I thought I could. Then we talked about the issue of salt. I confessed that I was a lifelong "salt-a-holic." We had a serious discussion about how the salt caused the body to retain fluid and put additional pressure on the heart. I resolved that day to do without table salt. She encouraged me to do those three things and then come back to see her in a month.

New energy stirred in me. I confronted my prayers from the month before. It had not been God's will for David to live and me to die. He intended, I could see ever more clearly, for me to live. And strongly the thought came from Him that day, *If I will for you to live, then you had better live well.* That meant coming to grips with my grief and doing something positive to fulfill God's purposes for permitting me to live. It meant keeping the food diary and living on 2,000 calories a day. It meant doing without table salt. So day by day, I did the three things she had asked me to do. By the next appointment, I had done as she had suggested, and when I weighed, I had lost weight. I began to believe that there was hope. I had to just keep doing the same thing. Mary somehow believed also, and she constantly encouraged me.

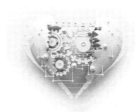

HOPE

Our thirty-ninth wedding anniversary approached in August. After our previous air-travel disaster, we were not up to the weariness of handling all the LVAD equipment going through an airport and onto a flight. We wanted to do something special, however. As energy and hope returned, we determined that we would do something. Then the idea came that we could drive thirty miles north of Denton to Gainesville and take the "Heartland Flyer" train to Oklahoma City. We had some points that could be used for a weekend at a downtown hotel there. And the travel was so easy. No metal detectors or long concourses.

We parked in a handicapped place at the train station in Gainesville just thirty feet from where the train stopped. The conductor just picked the heavy LVAD base unit off the walker and placed it on the train and folded up the walker. He rolled our bags on the train. All we had to do was walk to our seat. The train was not the fastest or most efficient means of travel, but it served our purposes. We didn't mind the little towns in Oklahoma where it stopped. And when we got to Oklahoma City, there was a cab waiting near where we got off. The cabbie loaded all the equipment, walker, and luggage into the trunk of the cab and took us the two blocks to our hotel. It was a four dollar cab ride, and I tipped the cabbie generously. At the hotel, a young bellman loaded all our items on a cart and took them to our hotel room. The desk people worked with us to have a room near the elevator to minimize walking distance. Our deal with the points included breakfast, so we were all set.

There was not much going on in Oklahoma City that weekend, so the young bellman offered to use the hotel van to drive us anywhere we wanted to go. He drove us to the location of the Oklahoma bombing, which was a few blocks away, that night. The next day, he drove us to a shopping mall. I am not much on shopping malls, but it been a very long time since we had been to a mall. I sat and read a book and Mary just slowly meandered, window shopping in one store after another. Doing these ordinary things contributed to the welling hope in us. We were having a nice time.

For our anniversary meal, we decided to go to the Mickey Mantle steakhouse in the heart of Bricktown. We dressed up a little to make it special. I was adept by now at dressing in such a way that the batteries and harness were not so obvious. There was nothing I could do about the noise of the LVAD, and people would look around to see where the noise was coming from. But amazingly, no one ever said anything, ever. This restaurant was baseball Mecca for me. I enjoyed all the photos on the wall of the "Mick," remembering my childhood days when he was my favorite baseball player. We had a great meal. We laughed and lingered with some dessert and coffee for Mary. I asked the waiter for the check. He told me quietly that someone across the room had paid for our dinner! We looked around and he pointed out a young couple. They were casually dressed. She had on a ball cap with a pony tail coming out the back of the cap. We thanked the waiter and decided we would stop at their table and say "thank you." We introduced ourselves and expressed our thanks. They were so open and cordial, and invited us to sit for a minute and chat with them. They told us that the joy that they saw in us across the room impressed them and they were moved to buy our meal. We shared our story briefly and explained about the noise of the LVAD. They were intrigued by it. As we were ready to leave, I mentioned that I believed that someday I would write a book. The young man grinned and handed me his business card. "Maybe I can help," he said. I looked at the card and saw that he was Ryan Tate, president of Tate Publishing Company. They were the 2006 Publisher of the Year for the Christian Storyteller's Association.

By the time we returned home, Rachel had begun to train for the White Rock Marathon in memory of David. She had the idea originally as a fundraiser for all the handicapped issues of the home remodeling and the van conversion to accommodate his wheel chair. She trained in the North Lakes area of Denton and I would meet her with water to encourage her. We had some special "Remembering Dave" shirts made up for all our family and friends. The preparation for this event continued throughout the fall.

SECTION III

LIVING WITH HEART #3

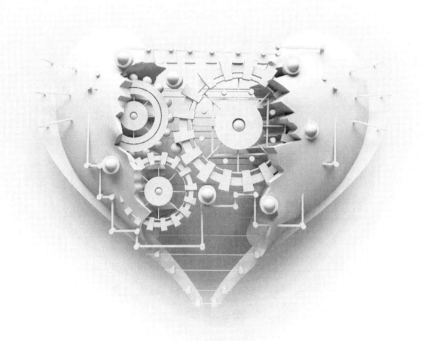

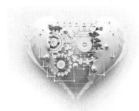

THE LVAD WEARS OUT

I made steady progress with my weight loss and looked forward to the monthly appointments with Dee Rollins. This was a long journey, but we were going the right direction and making progress. Meanwhile, I had a couple of red alarms on my LVAD controller that immediately went away when I reset them. I went to the heart failure clinic in September to have it checked out. Several tests were run and then my coordinator, Amy Boronow, explained that she would overnight the vent filter to the manufacturer. She called back two days later and reported that there were many metal flakes in the filter, indicting that the pump was wearing out. This was alarming and started the thinking of what to do next if the LVAD failed.

Dr. Meyer explained that in his scope of experience, there had not been an LVAD replacement with another LVAD. It was not out of the question, but if it came to that, it would be the first one that he had done. In short, it would mean replacing one bridge for another one. There was no assurance it would lead anywhere. The red alarms continued sporadically. I sent my vent filters frequently to be tested and the results showed an increase in the metal shavings, an indication that the pump was wearing out quickly. Now that I was losing weight steadily and was demonstrating the possibility of qualifying for a future heart transplant, serious consideration was given to the replacement. The insurance company would have to see all the data and agree to the replacement. It was another long serious surgery. There would again be a long vertical and shorter horizontal incision. I would be placed on a heart/lung machine, and then the old LVAD would be extracted. This could pose a problem, depending on how impeded it was with surrounding tissue. Once it was removed, Dr. Meyer would hook up a new LVAD and create a new hole in my stomach for the new drive-line. Dr. Meyer was ever encouraging, explaining it casually as if he were a mechanic just replacing the water pump on a vehicle. I was encouraged that the insurance company agreed. I asked Dr. Meyer what he did with the old LVAD when he took it out. He was surprised. "Do you want it?" he asked. Yes, I wanted it. I was going to write a book. He assured me that he would preserve it and give it to me.

On November 15, 2006, just two days shy of eighteen months since I had the first LVAD, I was wheeled in for the replacement surgery. Dr. Meyer thought since I was in better health than when I had the original LVAD, that I might be hospitalized for ten days to two weeks. Many of the issues were the same: lots of people were praying, and there was a difficult surgery ahead. Some issues were different: there were possible problems with extracting the LVAD, and there was the absence of my son from those praying and encouraging.

There was difficulty extracting the old LVAD, but finally the surgery was successfully completed. This time I was out of ICU quickly and amazingly, I was home in four days! I had worried that another Thanksgiving would be interrupted, but this was not so. The quick recovery and continued weight-loss buoyed my hopes for going on the transplant list in the future.

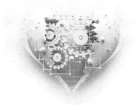

THE ROCK

The White Rock Marathon was scheduled for December 10, 2006. We had a wonderful turnout in support of Rachel. Dr. Meyer wore a "Remembering Dave" shirt and ran a half marathon. Some of our family and friends joined Rachel at various points in the twenty-six miles. We saw many of the "Remembering Dave Earp" shirts at a variety of places along the race route. Our charitable benefit focus was the Scottish Rite Children's Hospital. Mary and I had a chance to spend some time with some of the children the day before the marathon. My friend, Ray Pittman, pushed me in my wheelchair alongside Rachel the last mile. It was a great way to remember David. More than $10,000 was raised for the children of Scottish Rite. It was the largest individual fundraising effort of the "Rock."

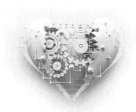

LIFE WITH THE LVAD

I was living a "new normal" life with the second LVAD. The dressing still had to be changed. The supplies had to be ordered. These tasks were an everyday part of Mary's schedule. Over time, the battery capacity diminished. When I had new batteries, and when they were fully charged, they would last four hours. Now, as the batteries aged, they often lasted less than two hours. I had to plan more carefully if I left the house and the security of being tethered to the LVAD base unit. The bag of spare batteries that I carried now always had to have at least six spare batteries. The bag loaded with the batteries and the manual pump weighed almost twenty pounds.

I longed for a shower. But I was alive, even with many complications. Tatum and A.J. would come into the bedroom to see me all "tethered" with my connection to the base unit. They loved removing and inserting the batteries into the base unit slots where they were recharged. I also used a "sleep machine" with a big mask that covered my face and helped my breathing when I slept at night. I was a sight, straight from a space movie with my mask on connected by a tube to the sleep machine and my LVAD controller hanging on me connected by the big tether to the base unit. And I was a sound too, the constant *swish, swish* of the pump noise emitting from the vent. This was normal life for

Grampsie and neither Tatum nor A.J. seemed in the least both-ered by it. When I sat in my chair in the den and the controller alarmed, indicating the batteries needed changing, I would ask one of them to go to the bedroom and get me some charged bat-teries. The batteries were almost heavier than their little bodies could carry, but they always wanted to help Grampsie.

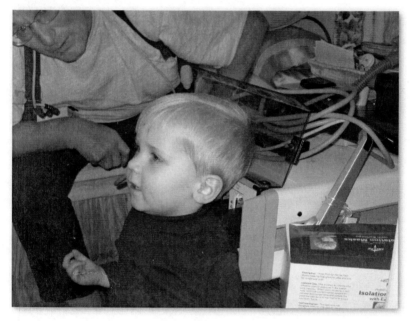

"New normal" – Governor leans over to hook up his batter-ies and disconnect from the base unit. A.J. is helping.

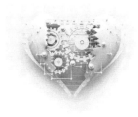

PROGRESS

When I had my appointment with Dee Rollins in late January, 2007, I celebrated with her. On that appointment in less than seven months, living with an LVAD and a replacement, I had lost almost eighty pounds!

I was now ready to begin the process at Baylor for qualifying for the transplant list. I would go through many tests in February, 2007, toward this purpose. I had to have a colonoscopy, various MRIs, an afternoon-long lung test to assure I had adequate lung capacity. I learned there was a transplant committee at Baylor that had to consider all the tests and approve me for a transplant. The approval of the committee was not a given. Although I had done well with the LVADs and made considerable progress with my health, I still had some issues. Some of the factors with my blood made me a difficult match. My body size was still a factor. I had an "eighteen-wheeler" body and would not be able to live with a "lawnmower motor." I could only have a heart from a large man. Most large men did not have good health. I would need an offensive lineman type donor. I heard of the "battles," of the back-and-forth discussion on the committee about whether I should be put on the transplant list. The other issue again was whether the insurance company would approve a heart transplant. The serious nutshell analysis was that no one wanted to waste a good organ on someone who was going to die anyway, and the insurance company sure did not want to pay unless there was some assurance that I might live successfully with a transplant.

This was a quickly moving time in our life. Tatum turned five and was looking forward to being in kindergarten. Rachel and Clint found out they were going to have Sadie in October. And DLynn shared with us her emerging desire and call to go to the seminary. She was considering taking a leave of absence from teaching. I was waiting to see if I would go on the transplant list.

In early March, with all the tests out of the way and waiting to hear if I would be put on the transplant list, Mary and I decided we would accept an invitation to a conference in the Washington D.C. area. We planned to go a few days early, as I wanted to make a trip up to Gettysburg again. We were running the risk of another disaster at an airport or on an airplane as had happened the previous March. This time we were in much better shape emotionally and physically and had extra time going and coming to allow plenty of rest and stress free movement through the security checks. We enjoyed our trips out away from Washington and our tours in the city. We visited the new World War II Memorial for the first time. Our group had dinner inside the Smithsonian Air and Space Museum. The conferences were great, and I followed my previous routine: arrive early, sit near the far end of the front row. There was no way to "mute" the noise of the LVAD, but no one ever asked where the noise was coming from or what the batteries, computer, wires, and harness were for. Until the last day and the next-to-last speaker who was Joe Colavito, a motivational speaker. He was to be followed by Bob Woodruff, Washington Post reporter from the Watergate story. Then the conference would be over.

Joe, obviously distracted by my LVAD noise, and not sure where it was coming from, moved to the opposite end of the stage area from where I was seated. He finished his presentation, wondering all the while if there was some microphone malfunction. As I walked through the line to meet him and shake his hand, Joe looked at me and said, "How are you?"

"I'm alive," I replied.

"Could I pray for you?" he said.

"Yes!" I said. Others nearby leaned in to listen—obviously curious, but on the other hand, none of them had been willing to ask. Joe wanted to talk, so we moved to a couch in the lobby. Joe was from Atlanta and was headed home that afternoon as well. I pulled my original LVAD from my bag and handed it to Joe. He couldn't believe he was holding in his hands a "heart" that had been in me for eighteen months. Mary was upstairs in our room getting packed up to leave so we could get to Reagan Airport to go back to Texas. Joe and I did not make it back to the final session. There was another couple who sat and listened, wanting to hear the story. I became quick friends with Joe. We prayed together in the lobby of the hotel. He was fascinated with what would happen to me. He would call to check on me, and later in the year, sent Mary a tree for her birthday. He was such an encourager, and still is. One of the first people Mary called the day I got my heart transplant fourteen months later was Joe.

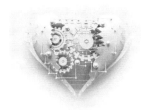

TRANSPLANT LIST

We got to Reagan airport with plenty of time to spare. As we sat waiting, I got an important call from Baylor. As of this day, March 14, 2007, I was officially being placed on the heart transplant list! The LVADs might really be a bridge to somewhere!

When we got back to Denton, we had to quickly readjust our lives. I could not travel farther than three hours from Dallas. If I got a transplant call, I needed to be at the hospital within three hours. My cell phone was to be the lifeline by which I would be contacted for a transplant. I had to keep it charged up and with me all the time.

Two weeks later I had an experience that confirmed the reasons for the rules. I was invited to speak at First Baptist Church in Belton, Texas. My friend Matt Nelson planned to drive me there as his parents were members of the church. Belton was just within the distance that I needed to maintain from Baylor Medical Center in Dallas in case a transplant call came. I had medical appointments in Dallas that morning that did not go quickly. By the time I got back to Denton and retrieved some extra batteries, Matt and I were late getting away. We had to drive through Fort Worth at rush hour and began to encounter such heavy rains that we could hardly see to drive. Fortunately, we were driving in "Big Red," Matt's diesel rig that barely cleared the growing pools of water on the interstate. We finally arrived at the church session almost an hour late. We missed the meal that was included in the event. I immediately began speaking about my experiences and the significance of the impact of prayer in my life, not realizing that very night that more prayer would be needed to get us home. We concluded a successful session, and got in "Big Red" to head home.

We stopped for coffee in Temple, and the lady who served us asked us which direction we were headed on the interstate. When we told her north, she shook her head and told us the severe flooding that direction had flooded the interstate. It was closed at a point about forty-five miles away and more than one hundred miles from home. We continued north on the interstate, trying to think of alternate routes in case it was still closed. However, in that part of Texas there are not any viable alternate routes to the interstate, so we continued with the hope that the interstate problems would be soon resolved. When we arrived at the traffic backup point, we pulled off the interstate to a convenience store. There were many people milling around full of rumor-type information. At this point, using what I had learned from the past, I change the mode from *auto* to *fixed*.

I talked to Clint on the cell phone. He was having a challenging night, serving as the family emergency coordinator. Rachel had flown to Miami for the prosecution of a case and was trying to fly back to DFW. She had called Clint and told him to find her a bus or some way to get home, since the airport was closed due to the weather. He was frantically trying to help Rachel with her emergency and me with mine and take care of A.J. all at the same time. He had talked to the sheriff in Hillsboro who had told him of an alternate route that might work that would require us to double back more than forty-five miles. I had brought more than enough batteries, I thought, for the length of our journey. But since I was in a hurry when I had gotten in with Matt before we left home, I had left my double backup bag in my car.

Finally we arrived at the alternate route, only to encounter a local volunteer fire department truck and a long line of traffic that had also tried the alternate route. This small state highway was now closed. Matt turned around, and I called Clint again regarding the only other possible alternate route, the other north/south interstate about fifty miles to the east. He had called the sheriff in Corsicana on that interstate and had been told it was closed in some areas. Matt and I decided that was our best option, anyway. We finally arrived in Corsicana and headed for the interstate entrance, only to encounter a fire truck blocking the entrance! We were told that entrance was closed, but that if we took the business interstate five miles south of town, we might be able to get on. So we did. We finally arrived at Matt's house almost four hours later than we would normally have. On fixed mode, I had gotten light-headed, but on this challenging night, we never had a red heart alarm!

Mary had to make a trip to Wellington in the spring, so I went with her as far as my boundary would allow. I stayed at a hotel in Wichita Falls the three days she was gone. My crazy sisters drove from Floydada to stay at the same hotel and take care of their little brother, standing by to take me to Dallas in case of a heart transplant call.

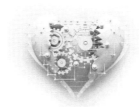

WORK-RELATED CHALLENGE

In June, 2007, a work deadline loomed with the NASD regarding my licensing. The NASD has a standing requirement that to maintain my securities registration I complete a half day recertification every three years. July 1, 2007, was the deadline for this three year period. I had never had to go to a secure testing center before with the LVAD. It takes some time to get set up to do this certification, and I had initiated the paperwork in April and paid the required fee, not wanting to press the deadline too closely. The day after the Memorial Day holiday I was scheduled to do my session at the Thompson Prometrics testing center in Dallas. There is a very specific list of things you must be sure to have with you. You must bring a photo ID and registration paperwork, and you absolutely must be on time. At the beginning of the process, you are fingerprinted.

Before the session begins, you have to place everything in your pockets in a secure locker: wallet, cell phone, calculators, papers, keys, pens … *everything*. I realized only at that moment that I had a dilemma. Even though I had just put in fresh batteries, there was a good possibility that my batteries would have to be changed during the three hours. And I was on the heart transplant list, so it was imperative that I have my cell phone with me. And I was supposed to keep my manual pump with me at all times. If you have never been to one of these busy testing-centers, there is a continual litany of requests. For example, some might plead that their session allows a special calculator or they are sick today and need extra time. The testing director and the testing monitor are hard core...there are no exceptions. Thus my reluctance to bring up my situation, but of course, I had to.

After my explanation about the LVAD and the equipment needs, I was quickly told that no matter what I said there would be no exceptions. I quickly considered my options. I absolutely had to have the certification to continue to operate my business after July 1, 2007. There was a possibility that the batteries would make it, and even if they did alarm, I could turn the alarm off and continue the session. And though I was supposed to have the manual pump with me at all times, I had never had to use it in an emergency. So, I decided that I would store all the stuff and then came back to the front desk for my fingerprinting. I waited quite a long time and then the testing director walked over to me and said rather directly "Does that *thing* have a volume control? Can you turn it down for us?" I explained that it did not have a volume control and that the noise was just the consequence of how it worked. So she had me be seated and walked away.

Again I waited a very long time.

Finally, the testing center director brought the testing monitor along with her, and she explained that the noise of the LVAD would be too distracting to all the other people being tested and therefore, I would not be allowed to do my session. Then she handed me a piece of paper with an 800 telephone number on it and told me that I should call that number and they would work on some accommodations for my problem. I was not only surprised, but I was angered. The individual testing cubicles at the center are all equipped with headphones and there seemed to be no likelihood of distraction to me. I objected, knowing that my deadline would be looming soon. If it was difficult getting a regular session scheduled, how difficult would it be to get a "special session" scheduled? She was hearing none of my objections. She just repeatedly said in response to everything I said, "Have a nice day." The waiting room of the testing center was absolutely quiet, as everyone watched to see what would happen.

So I sat down on the front row opposite the fingerprinting station and dialed the 800 number I was given. It rang many times, no answer. I redialed and this same thing happened over and over. In frustration, I called my firm's compliance officer and he was also shocked at what was happening. He explained that the handicapped laws were being violated.

I went back to the testing director and told her that there was no answer to the 800 number after being tried repeatedly, and there was contact underway from my firm to NASD regarding the fact that my required session was being denied. The testing director simply replied, "Just keep trying. Have a nice day." So I advised her that I would not leave without something in writing signed by her indicating that she was denying my session. She replied, "I'm not writing or signing anything!"

My frustration had reached a breaking point. I am a very tall man, and I just stood immediately in front of the sign in the area so that anyone coming into the center would have to stand in line behind me. Then I told her that I was not leaving that point until I had her business card and the contact information for her management. She was the testing center manager so I knew there was no one "higher up" at this location. She looked at me, and I didn't budge. So she went inside and consulted with the monitor and came back and gave me her business card that also had the phone number for the regional manager. I left, having killed a day without accomplishing anything. A man followed me out the door to talk to me, sure that there would likely be a lawsuit out of the episode. He said, "I saw what happened and will testify for you if you need me." He gave me his business card.

That episode began a two-week-long litany of conference calls with firm lawyers, personnel with NASD, and counsel with Thompson Prometric. I advised that I knew that the testing was a requirement but I wanted an alternate site so that I did not have to deal with the same personnel. I would have to get a refund from that testing center and then try to get scheduled with a different one.

The only one I could get that gave me any time buffer required me to be at the testing center near the busiest intersection in Dallas for an 8 a.m. session on a Monday morning, meaning that I really needed to arrive by 7:30 a.m. One of the reasons that it was so difficult to schedule was that now, because of my LVAD, it was deemed that my session had to be conducted and monitored in a private room. Many testing centers do not have those kinds of accommodations. When I arrived for this session I was met at the door by an official who immediately began explaining that there had been a problem downloading their software and no testing would take place that day! So began a frantic effort to get rescheduled. It was like starting from scratch, and by then there was only a slot left late on the last Saturday afternoon in June—much too close to the deadline.

I spent several days calling back and forth. NASD wanted to know why I had not taken the second scheduled session and didn't seem to grasp that the testing center had been closed for the day due to the software download problem. I spoke to six different people over three days with NASD and with the testing firm.

Finally, late in the evening on Thursday, June 21, I was on the phone, talking to the testing center person who had promised to call me back and seemed to have compassion on me. We discussed all the possibilities. I asked if I could drive to Waco or Tyler or Oklahoma City. None of those testing centers had a private room. I asked her what I was going to do. There seemed to be no option. I asked her if there were any other metroplex centers that had a private room. She said the one in Bedford did and looked at their schedule and saw that they were booked for the remainder of June. Then she said, "It looks like if you could make it there at 7 a.m. tomorrow morning, they could work you in." I quickly agreed to take that slot, even though I had a long drive and no familiarity of where that testing center was located.

After a short night, I got up very early to be sure that I found the testing center to be on time. When I arrived on time the lady who greeted me had been called by the lady who had worked out the time the night before and was very kind and helpful. She verified all my paperwork, fingerprinted me, and led me to the private room which has a window so the monitor can be sure that all the rules are followed. How grateful I was to complete the requirement before noon and be on my way! This entire process, normally taking someone only a three-hour session on one day, had taken me more than a month.

By now, DLynn was excited to be enrolled at Dallas Theological seminary in their Master's degree program. She was already taking classes. In June she had been asked to be the part-time women's ministry coordinator at our church. She earned enough from her part time job that she and Tatum could manage financially, although their cash flow would be tight.

In July, Mary went to her usual Kelley reunion in Collingsworth County. I went as far as Wichita Falls, and Mary left me in a hotel there. Since I would be alone, I had verified that if I got a transplant call, there was a taxi service in Wichita Falls that guaranteed to get me to Dallas in three hours. Tatum was with us and went on to the reunion with Mary. I was dissatisfied with the hotel where I was staying. The room was dirty, the TV was broken, and no one seemed interested in resolving the issues. I was alone, with nothing to do, so I got on the phone and checked around to see if I could find a better place. I was surprised that another, better place offered me such a great deal! I called the cab company that had arranged to transport me to Dallas if I needed a heart transplant. The company quickly sent a cabbie to load my equipment and take me to the other hotel. This place, the Howard Johnson Park Plaza Hotel, appealed to me with the wide variety of possible activities. I discussed with the management hosting a new reunion for our family every Labor Day weekend. I made the arrangements and plans while staying there. We would have the first Labor Day Family Fun Weekend in 2007, only six weeks later.

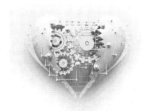

FIRST TRANSPLANT CALL

We had only been back in Denton ten days when we got our first heart transplant call. We couldn't believe it! Mary and I had just left the mall area and the transplant coordinator called and said to get home and get our things together and they would call back in a little while. By 8 p.m. we were loaded up. The call came and we were on our way to Dallas to have a heart transplant! DLynn rode with us and as I sped down the HOV lane, she said, "I can't believe you are driving yourself to have a heart transplant!" Rachel and Clint made arrangements for A.J. and joined us on tenth floor Roberts, where I was being prepped. About midnight they all followed as the nurses rolled my bed to the elevator then down to the operating room on the second floor. I lay waiting in an open area in front of the operating room door. I was ready. We waited and waited. Then Dr. Meyer came out and said that it was not going to happen. The doctor who had harvested the matching heart had called immediately when he saw the heart physically and could actually see that the heart had damages that were severe enough to keep the heart from being useable. What an emotional letdown that was! We had called all our family and everyone's hopes were up. The nurse on the tenth floor asked if we wanted to just stay the night and go home later in the morning. We didn't. We were home by 4 a.m., exhausted and just as emotionally down as we had been high just a few hours before. I had to adjust my attitude that if the transplant were to happen, it would be at the right time. Life is about never giving up.

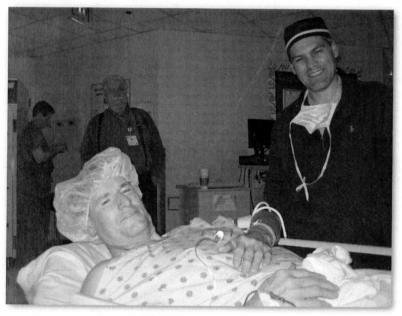

"Dress rehearsal" – waiting for a heart transplant that didn't happen

On August 13, 2007, Mary and I celebrated our fortieth anniversary. Rachel called us and said she had arranged something special to help us celebrate our anniversary: a hot-air balloon ride! She picked us up at our house and drove us thirty miles to McKinney by 6 a.m. The hot-air balloon lifted off just at sunrise and we quietly floated over a portion of Collin County. Of course, we had our black bag with us that contained extra batteries and the manual pump. I also had my cell phone just in case I got another heart transplant call. I mused about how many other people had taken their LVAD and the equipment necessary on a hot-air balloon ride.

I was already on a different kind of ride: another LVAD failure roller coaster. About the time of this special anniversary, I began having occasional unexplained LVAD alarms. This LVAD was now nine months old. The other, more troubling, issue was that I began to get out of breath if I did anything strenuous. There were moments when my head would spin as in the worst heart failure days.

Labor Day weekend, 2007, marked the fulfillment of one of my purposes for living. Our family celebrated the first annual Family Fun Weekend at the Howard Johnson Plaza Hotel in Wichita Falls. There were almost forty of us for the weekend. We had a great time sharing, singing, playing games, swimming, and remembering. I so enjoyed watching the little children run around the indoor putting-green. On Sunday night there was a special fireworks celebration just outside our hotel. Wichita Falls had had a major flood earlier in the year that had forced the cancellation of their annual July Fourth fireworks show. We were blessed as a family that the show had been rescheduled for Labor Day weekend. As many of us made the long walk to the back exit of the hotel to watch the fireworks, I had to stop and catch my breath several times. The LVAD journey is a constantly challenging one. I clearly understood why it was a "bridge" and not an end solution.

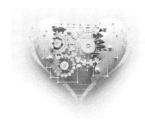

FAILING LVAD

Soon the LVAD was pumping at 120 beats a minute even on *auto* mode. I prayed even more urgently for a transplant. Mary has been the source of great impact at the most strategic moments of my life. As we worried, one day while she was changing the dressing, she said to me, "You may not have the transplant until you get the book written." The book that she referred to is one that we had been collaborating on for a few months. We had now lived successfully with two LVADs for almost two and a half years. Our friends at the Baylor heart failure clinic and on the tenth floor of Roberts had seen that we had gained many practical insights on living with an LVAD. I was frequently asked to share my experiences with someone who was in severe heart failure. Mary was also asked questions about how to care for someone in my condition. The literature about the LVAD had been very technical and scary for me. I wished that I had something very practical and day-to-day to prepare me and prepare Mary for what we faced when we came home with the LVAD. It had become clear to us that we were the ones to produce such a book. It could not be the kind of book that was published for wide reading. It had to focus on those who were in serious heart failure and for whom the LVAD might be a bridge. I had now lived two and half years without taking a shower! How is that possible? Our story was needed to help others know those kinds of things.

Mary's nudge made me grind away at night, committed to finishing the book. For it to be really practical, it needed lots of "how-to" pictures. We took almost a complete day and Mary made pictures of every aspect of the LVAD. She made pictures of me hooking up and connecting to the base unit and then to the batteries. She made pictures of our bathroom and how we had arranged a chair and a "handicapped" end to the shower head so that I could sit at the edge of tub and get clean without a shower and without risking an electrical problem with the wires and batteries. We decided to include funny stories to lighten the very serious issue of needing and dealing with an LVAD. I explained what it was like being the "Governor." I included a funny story about one late night incident. I was able to stretch the tether through the bathroom and into my office where I worked on my computer and studied my Bible. I was using a cane at his point because of the problem with the LVAD. As I came back through the bathroom, I lost my balance and fell backward into the bathtub with my feet sticking into the air. As I tried to figure how to get out, Mary sleepily came past me to use the commode. "What are you doing?" she said. I told her I fell into the bathtub. She started laughing. She finished, passed by me, and patted me on the head as she went back to the bedroom. She didn't even offer to help me! The next thing I knew, she had taken a picture of me! No thanks to her, while she laughed, I finally managed to use my cane to pull myself up and out of the tub. Many family and friends have laughed at the picture of the Governor in the bathtub.

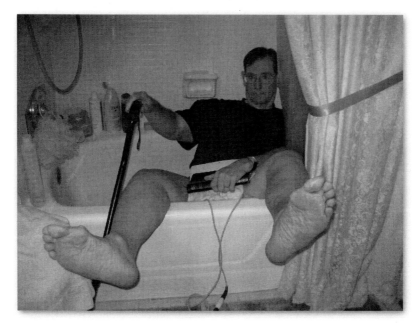

Governor in the tub

We completed this 130 page "how-to" book in late October, 2007. It was titled "Living Joyfully with an LVAD." I made arrangements with the local Kinko's to have 100 copies printed up. The Kinko's manager was interested in the story and understood that it was for a good cause, so he did the project at his cost. As soon as they were printed, Kinko's shipped them to Dallas to Baylor for me so that the staff in the heart failure clinic would each have one and all the nurses for every shift on tenth floor Roberts would have one. I also provided a supply for any patients who the staff thought might benefit from the book.

The completion of the book coincided with the birth of our third grandchild, Sadie Catherine Knowles, on October 26, 2007. What a joy to have a little baby in our family again! The joy was mixed with the revelation of the discovery of the source of the LVAD problem. The valve at the front end of the LVAD, where the blood came into it from the natural heart, was the problem. The valve was not opening fully, so despite the fact that the LVAD was pumping 120 times a minute, its true functionality was only about 35 percent. That meant that I was getting the equivalent of forty-two pumps a minute. My body was blood-starved due to the dysfunctional LVAD.

Encouragement comes from a variety of sources. Jim Kuykendall, a man in Denton who goes to our church and whom I had known for many years, had a heart transplant several years before. He came to my home to visit one afternoon. We cried and shared about his experience and the donor whose life was lost for Jim's heart. Jim had sat on an Easter Sunday afternoon in his backyard, thinking to himself that the transplant call would never come. That night he got the call. I was encouraged by Jim's visit.

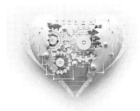

WAITING PATIENTLY

As the year 2007 ended, we prayed earnestly that a heart transplant would come soon. But it didn't. The rapid pumping of the LVAD shook my insides. Often my teeth chattered. I experienced a decline in functionality and energy. My head was dizzy due to the inadequate blood supply. I lived the roller-coaster effect in my emotions. Mary and I talked soberly about the truth that some people did not live long enough to have a transplant. One benefit of the problem was that it moved me to the very top of the transplant list. The transplant list is a complicated thing and was hard to understand. If a heart was available, who would get it? I learned that those who were dying in ICU were at the top of the list. Although I was not in ICU, I was considered in this category.

One day I asked Dr. Kuiper what would happen if the LVAD totally quit. He offered me the option of coming into the hospital into ICU and waiting there until a heart transplant came. But how long might that be? I recalled that a man that I had encouraged several years before who needed an LVAD had his LVAD fail within a few months. When I was awaiting my LVAD replacement on November 15, 2006, he had been waiting for weeks in ICU for a heart transplant. Miraculously, a heart came that very night. Dr. Meyer did his heart transplant that night and the very next morning did my LVAD replacement. I did not want to go into ICU for an indefinite period of time.

So many people had prayed for me for so long. I could see and hear their discouragement and, in some cases, anger with God for not answering this prayer. I had been praying for a long time for the family of the heart donor and the grief they would be experiencing if I did get a transplant. My granddaughter, Tatum, now six years old and about to finish kindergarten, showed great understanding one day. She said to me very seriously, "Grampsie, it will be sad for you to get a heart transplant." I told her no, that it would be a joyful answer to prayer. Then she replied so seriously, "No, Grampsie, it will be sad, because someone has to die for you to get a heart transplant." Her wisdom came from real-life experience. Our heartfelt conversations have led to another desire of my heart that I have asked God for. Tatum and I talk about her wedding day at some point in the future. I have asked God to allow me to live long enough to walk her down the aisle, and then have a dance with her in her wedding dress. I believe I will live to see that day. Time will tell.

By May 7, 2008, I had lived almost three years with an LVAD. Considering all the issues and complications, that was pretty amazing. What had started out to be a bridge had become a very long bridge. But the bridge was going out quickly. In the nick of time, it seemed, I got a call from the transplant center. There was a heart and it was somewhere in the area. How quickly could I get to Dallas? This, in many respects, was a repeat of the night more than nine months before when I got the first call. I was there and prepped. Dr. Shelley Hall was covering for Dr. Kuiper. I knew her well, as she and Dr. Kuiper were the two heart failure cardiologists who had treated me these more than three years. She said confidently to Mary and me, "This is going to happen. There is only a remote chance, less than five percent, that it won't happen." Wow, how our hopes were buoyed!

It seemed certain as I lay in the OR with an IV in my jugular vein. For sure it was going to happen! Then Dr. Meyer was over me, looking into my face. "Mr. Earp, it is not going to happen tonight." I thought he was kidding. He wasn't. He explained that the heart was a perfect match. But when it was harvested and the doctor touched one of the heart veins, it crunched. The veins were so loaded with plaque and blockage that they crunched! It was a perfect match, but I didn't need a damaged heart.

It was so late we decided to stay in the room on tenth floor Roberts and go home later in the day. But the process languished, the shift changed and no one seemed to know what to do with a patient who almost had a transplant but didn't. I was angry and wanted to go home. There was some kind of paper snafu that resulted in me lying in a bed for hours waiting to go home but unable to be "officially" released. It was a frustrating emotional exclamation point on the transplant that wasn't. It was after noon before we left Baylor. Once we were home, I saw that this wild roller coast ride had taken a huge toll on Mary. She was back to the "take care of the LVAD" mode, and she was exhausted after loading and unloading all the equipment once again. We both needed a break.

SECTION IV

LIVING WITH HEART #4

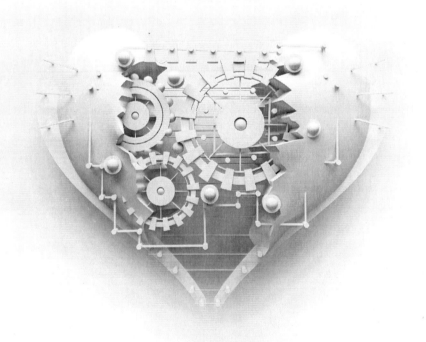

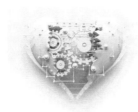

ANOTHER DRESS REHEARSAL?

Mary and I made plans to take a break just a few days later on May 14. I encouraged her to get away for a few hours on her own and do something she enjoyed. The Texas Rangers were playing an afternoon baseball game scheduled to start at 1 p.m. I talked Clint into taking the afternoon off and taking A.J. and me to the baseball game in Arlington. When I talked to him early that morning, I told him to come to the house and back up to the garage and load up my wheelchair. At 9:30 a.m. Amy Boronow, my transplant coordinator, called and told me not to get my hopes up, but that there might be a heart. It was like the little boy crying "wolf" to me. I explained I was going with my grandson to the baseball game and I didn't want to disappoint him. "Okay," she said. Things did not appear to be moving quickly, if at all. But she emphasized that I keep my cell phone with me and that it be on and charged up. I sat on my bed and filled my bag with batteries. I was ready to go to the baseball game. It would be a nice distraction. The "nacho kid" called and said that he and A.J. were on the way and to be ready. I could tell he was excited to go the game, or was it the nachos? I had barely hung up the phone when Amy Boronow called back. She told me that this heart situation was moving a little more quickly and I needed to come on to Baylor, although the timeframe was not yet urgent. I didn't want to disappoint the boys headed for the baseball game, so I made a quick decision. I called the "nacho kid" back and told him that when he pulled up behind my house to not load the wheelchair, but to come inside where I was in the bedroom. Within ten minutes he and A.J. breezed and in and wondered what was up. I explained to him that he needed to load the LVAD base unit and all the equipment in my jeep. He and A.J. needed to do this for me and then go on to the baseball game. I was not about to disappoint the boys. The equipment was quickly loaded, and they were off to the baseball game. I headed to Dallas, alone, in my jeep. When I was driving through Lewisville, about a half hour from Baylor, I got another call from Amy, wanting to know where I was. I told that I was in Lewisville on my way, driving myself with all my equipment. She couldn't believe it! "Please, Amy, just have some people meet me in the Hamilton Heart Hospital parking lot with some carts for all my equipment and a wheelchair for me." A half hour later, I pulled into the parking lot. On cue, three of the heart failure staff ran to my jeep, pushing a wheelchair and two carts for all the equipment. Another ten minutes and they had me in a room on tenth floor Roberts. I thought about the baseball saying: three strikes and you're out! Or it would be more encouraging to think "the third time's a charm?"

I had, as nonchalantly as possible, left a couple of voicemails for Mary, knowing that she was not expecting to hear from me. She was not answering, but at the moment the situation did not appear to be urgent.

I was told that the possible heart was local and that it would be at least a couple of hours before anything further happened. Mary called and I told her where I was and what was happening. She delayed as if doing so might make this the real performance and not just another dress rehearsal. She and DLynn came a couple of hours later.

As I lay in the bed waiting, I got a call on my cell phone that was out of left field. A long battle had been waged over several months to get my long-term disability coverage to begin paying. It had taken forever, complicated by the fact that claims people far away over the telephone could not understand how I had lived with a mechanical pump for three years and had just filed for long-term disability at the beginning of the year. Why not three years before? "Easy," I had said. "Three years ago I thought I was going to die and was preparing for a death claim on my life insurance." Joe Mahoney, my firm's managing director, had made calls on my behalf and had e-mailed a picture of me with the LVAD. It astounded me that after all the time and frustration, this call finally came this afternoon, as I lay waiting on a heart transplant. It was from the claims person with the disability insurance company. He apologized for the long delay, told me the claim had been approved, and that disability payments would begin on Friday!

By 7 p.m. Dr. Kuiper told us that it looked like it was going to happen, but it might be 9 or 10 p.m. All our family had gathered at Baylor once again. While we waited, during some on going speculations about the donor, I had a huge misunderstanding. I took seriously my sister's teasing remarks that the donor was a large "preacher." Somehow I locked in on that as fact, and it took Mary some serious convincing that it was a joke. Truthfully, no one knew anything about the donor. I had asked Dr. Kuiper about the donor. He said, "You don't want to know." I wondered what he meant. Was he speaking generally that no matter whom it was, I didn't want to know, or was he speaking specifically with knowledge that I was not allowed to know of some horrible death? As I pondered the question, I prayed once again for the family of the donor.

Time passed, and I encouraged everyone waiting to go to the cafeteria and get something to eat. At 9 p.m., Dr. Kuiper said it looked like it might be midnight before the transplant happened. At 11 p.m., he explained that there was an operating room scheduling problem, and the transplant would be scheduled for 8:30 the next morning. Mary, DLynn, Rachel, and Clint got two rooms at the hotel just up the street.

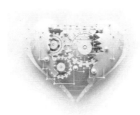

TRANSPLANT

The word was spread quickly that at 8:30 a.m., Thursday, May 15, 2008, I would have a heart transplant at A. Webb Roberts Hospital, by now a very familiar place. The next morning my family was in my room and walked down with me to the operating room one more time. They were joined by a waiting room filled with our pastor and many other family and friends. I went into the OR, and I carefully instructed Dr. Meyer that I wanted the second LVAD and, if it was possible, I wanted a picture of the worn out natural heart when it was removed. He agreed to my request, if it was possible. He said Dr. Ring would try to use his cell phone to take a picture of the natural heart. Dr. Meyer and I had discussed collaborating on a book previously. I told him before they put me under that I wanted a picture of all four hearts for my book. He put me under.

Hours passed in the waiting room while the visitors talked. Melvin Jones, a volunteer and heart transplant veteran, came to sit with our family. He had come and waited a long time with us the night before. His heart transplant had been almost five years earlier. A screen in the waiting room showed the progress of the surgery. When the LVAD was successfully out, the news was reported to Amy by a call from the OR. Now that the LVAD was out, Amy and Mary carried out a ritual in the waiting room.

Amy held a trash can and Mary ceremoniously threw the batteries and the manual pump into the trash can. When the news was shared that the transplant had been successfully completed, I am told that a great time of cheering and rejoicing was had by all. In the middle of the afternoon, Dr. Meyer arrived to the waiting room and shared that all had gone well.

There was a glow in my body when I woke up. It felt good. Finally my body was getting enough blood. My mind was clear. There were no cobwebs, no hallucinations. The pain was not bad. I bordered on laughing out loud with celebration! Soon, Mary came in and kissed me. She said Dr. Ring was sitting at a table nearby and told her that I was doing well. Everyone in the waiting room appeared briefly, in spite of the ICU rules.

I determined not to spend long in the ICU. The next morning Dr. Meyer told me that I needed to sit up that day. So if sitting up was good, in my thinking sitting up all afternoon was better. I almost wore myself out sitting up before someone got me back in bed. The quietness stunned me. I had been so used to the pump sensation in my body and the noise of the LVAD that I just soaked up the quiet solitude. Were they really gone? Yes!

The ICU was a collection of the most challenging cases. The man directly across from me from Lewisville, Texas, was younger than me but appeared much older. His lungs had been ruined by an asbestos-related career. He had just received two new, pink lungs. His double lung transplant replaced two lungs that literally fell apart during the transplant. A man opposite me was not with it and obviously needed the treatment intended. He was not willing to give his consent. Round and round the process went; one family member called another, and then that one would come to the room to try to convince him to give his consent. He never did while I was in ICU. As with many people who were going through their own valleys of death, once I was gone from their presence, I did not know what happened to them.

By the second day I was lobbying with Dr. Shelley Hall to let me move up to tenth floor Roberts. Shelley was on in place of Johannes Kuiper. As we discussed my move, the ICU nurse began to look for a place to put in a backup IV for the transfer, because Baylor protocol now required one. She seemed very concerned about the Baylor protocol. I asked Shelley Hall if that was really necessary. I was doing great and was tired of being stuck over and over. Why stick me for backup? Dr. Capeheart was at the bedside of the patient one bed over. He had been involved with our family on many occasions, dealing with PICC lines for David on multiple occasions. He often had looked in on me when I was on tenth floor Roberts. He had a reputation there of appearing in the middle of the night when the night nursing staff ordered pizza. He loved pizza. Shelley had been bantering back and forth with Dr. Capeheart. She looked over and asked him, "John, what do you think? How about we just say 'to hell with the Baylor protocol' and not stick Mr. Earp again?" He looked back at her and said, "Shelley, just do what you think is best." Shelley looked the nurse in the eye and said, "Don't put the IV in." The nurse was coming unglued that on her watch, this was happening. I was ecstatic.

I had a wonderful few days on tenth floor Roberts. I loved my young, Russian nurse, Vadim. I was fascinated by his story. A young tech came by my room often to see if I needed anything. He kept me supplied with popsicles, cheese, and crackers. I had lots of visitors. Many of them were staff people who had read the LVAD book that we had provided everyone on the floor. I was up and walking the tenth floor oval soon. I went home the seventh day. There were no machines, no doctors going with me to instruct anybody, just Mary and me, a lot of medication, and a new protocol to follow.

Home felt a lot different. The LVAD cabinet disappeared from our bedroom. I was moving on with the life that I had been given. Don't be fooled into thinking there were no issues. There were many. I started out taking sixty pills a day. I had to track and record my blood pressure, and stick my finger three times a day to check my blood sugar. The big issue was avoiding infection and avoiding rejection. I wore a mask over my face for the first ten days, all the time. If I had any exposure to the public, I would "mask up." For the first time in my life, I was constantly washing my hands. I did everything I could possibly do to avoid rejection.

The medication issue was daunting. I was on three anti-rejection drugs, plus many other pills. One of the anti-rejection drugs was cyclosporine. David had been on cyclosporine, and it smells to high heaven. Each individual pill is packed separately because when it is opened, a bad, skunk-like odor pervades the room. Finally I began on a very large dosage of prednisone, with it gradually being reduced over time. I took pills morning, noon, and night. And these pills were not cheap. It worries me every time I think about the cost of these vital medications. I repeated my earlier rehab regimens, walking in circles with the walker on the driveway and using hand weights to gain strength and endurance.

I had been home for two weeks and decided to go to Tatum's kindergarten graduation at our church. It was such a blessing. Of course I was "masked up" and sat outside the classroom during the party after the graduation. We went home and I had terrible trouble sleeping. I sat in my office at 4 a.m.; my gut burned with pain. I knew something was wrong. As soon as Mary got up, I told her that I had a problem. Having just jumped in the car and headed to Baylor on so many occasions over so many years, I resisted doing that. I was sick in my gut, throwing-up all over the bedroom throughout the day. When Mary called the heart failure center, we were told not to come, that this too would pass. It didn't, and by the next morning, we were panicky enough to load up and go to Baylor. We did the whole protocol: blood work, temperature, blood pressure, X-ray. The doctors sent us back to Denton, where I continued to throw-up. Our room started to reek with the odor of the throw-up. I was getting weaker, too. Late in the day, one of the heart failure staff called and said the X-ray showed a bowel obstruction and we needed to get to Baylor right away.

Mary called Clint to drive us and told him to drive as fast as he could. I could feel myself going down, and the light around me became dull and shaded. I was on the verge of passing out. Clint drove, and Mary called the police departments and the highway patrols as we blew through their jurisdictions. We were at Baylor in no time, and turned into the drive in front of Roberts Hospital. Clint tried to get me out into my wheelchair, but I passed out before he got me in it. As he was trying to hold me, the wheelchair started rolling away toward the ER. A couple of guys dressed in scrubs caught it and came running toward me with it. In a few seconds I was in the chair and they were running me down to the ER. My view of the Baylor ER is that it is a great place to get lost. These two guys repeatedly tried to get a blood pressure, but couldn't get one. After quick collaboration, with the understanding that I was a very recent heart-transplant patient, I was on my way up the elevator to tenth floor Roberts where Vadim began to try to get a blood pressure. He tried over and over. Finally he got one: sixty-two over thirty-eight! In a matter of minutes, there was a tube down my nose and the most awful brown bile liquid spewed through the tube to the gallon-size container, which had to be emptied over and over. In just one hour, almost 5,000 milliliters of the nasty bile had come out. I was made NPO, which means no food or drink, and this lasted six days. Constant X-rays were taken to determine the status of the obstruction. Mary has a strong sense of discernment and she wondered if I didn't have pneumonia. Dr. Black, one of the lung doctors, walked by, and she asked him to take a look. Sure enough one of the gut X-rays extended high enough for him to see my lungs, and yes, I did have pneumonia! The next three days was a terrific battle for me. On Saturday night, I thought I was dying and called Clint to bring Mary back down to Dallas. I had a very emotional night that night. On Sunday, Dr. Lamont finally allowed me a little ice, but nothing like a Popsicle. My attitude was terrible in the morning. I was ready for the tube to come out so I could eat and drink.

On Sunday evening, the quietness of the weekend settled in on tenth floor Roberts. There were seriously ill patients in all the rooms. One I know of died a few days later. The halls were quiet and there was a skeleton staff. My mouth was cracked and dry, bleeding. But my soul was soothed. I had channel-surfed on the TV and had found an old Gaither program that had some beautiful hymns. The door to my room was open, so I turned up the volume as loud as it would go. The rich beautiful music wafted down the hallway. I closed my eyes and listened. Those in other rooms listened too, the stress and worry of what would happen to them soothed over for a few minutes by these timeless hymns. The program stopped, and I turned off the TV. I heard perfect quietness in all the halls. The whole tenth floor Roberts, patients and staff, were inspired by hymns in the night. I prayed for God's abiding presence in each room. Monday came. Dr. Lamont concluded the blockage was cleared, and pulled the tube. I enjoyed Popsicles and Jell-o. I was able to walk on Tuesday, and was released on Wednesday morning.

The heart transplant had some unusual and unexpected physical effects on me. While I was still in the hospital, Mary noticed that I had a bad sore in my scalp. Dr. Kuiper looked at it, and had no explanation for the cause of it. It persisted. When I went to my barber Karmann Evans, he noticed it right away. For almost six months after the transplant, this open spot on my scalp persisted. Gradually it covered over, but there is still an abnormality in my hair at that spot. There has never been an explanation.

I have always sweated profusely. But for the five years prior to the transplant this sweating got worse. If I wore a suit, when I got home the shirt and suit would be soaked with sweat. When I spoke or taught in front of a group, those listening worried about the perspiration on me. I often carried two handkerchiefs to mop my brow. The transplant somehow totally changed my body thermometer. I am constantly cold, even in the summer. When I sit in my chair in the den, I usually have a blanket draped over me. I have not perspired a single time since the transplant!

Finally, with all the clips and stitches removed, the day came for me to have the long-awaited shower. It had been more than three years. One afternoon I took my time and sat on a chair, in the tub, with the shower running. I sat in the water almost an hour, savoring the moment, not wanting to get out. Later my friend, Bill Gasch, joked that the water pressure on his side of town almost went away while I was taking my shower.

I wanted very much to have a significant "celebration of life" after the heart transplant. Arrangements were made for a block of 400 tickets to the Texas Rangers game on Monday night, July 7. I invited as many of the nurses and staff from tenth floor Roberts and the heart failure clinic as could come. I invited all the doctors and their families to come. I invited friends, family, and many in our church. So many came that a few more tickets had to be purchased at the last minute for the extras who showed up. I was invited to share the job of throwing out the first pitch with Ronald McDonald. Tatum and A.J. enjoyed waiting for the moment in the same room underneath the stadium with Ronald McDonald. By 5 p.m. that day, Channel 11, Channel 4, and Channel 21 had new crews at the ballpark, talking to me, to our family, and to the doctors. The purpose in the evening was to raise the awareness so that people would make the effort to be signed up to be an organ donor. The story was the lead story that night on both Channel 4 and Channel 11.

Each week I gained a little ground. Late in July I wanted our family to go to Beaver's Bend for a couple of days. I paddled a canoe in the river, and rode the bumper boats with the grandchildren. We all ate purple snow cones that turned our tongues purple.

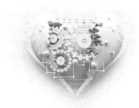

YANKEE STADIUM

I had still been holding on to a request that I had made of Dr. Meyer and Dr. Kuiper right after the heart transplant. This was the last year that baseball would be played in historic Yankee stadium, and I wanted to go. They had said maybe, but only after three months. I pressed a "yes" out of them. On August 13, Clint, A.J., and "the Governor" flew from DFW to Boston to spend two days there and visited Fenway Park to watch the Red Sox beat the Rangers badly twice. We did a little touring around Boston and then flew to New York City to see the Yankees play the Royals in Yankee stadium. When we arrived at the stadium, it was raining and looked like the game would be delayed or canceled. We were joined there by David's long-time friend, Todd Schietroma, who lives in a rural area about thirty miles from New York. We were fortunate to find shelter under one of the overhangs for the long wait. Finally, the decision was made to play the game. The Royals beat the Yankees in the ninth inning, scoring the winning runs off Mariano Rivera. The "nacho kid" was ecstatic! I enjoyed going to Yankee Stadium, but I wished for the old days when baseball was not played by millionaires. I wondered how many home runs that "T-Bone" Miller of the Lamesa Lobos would have hit in Yankee Stadium. We had a short night's sleep and then caught a flight back to Dallas the next morning.

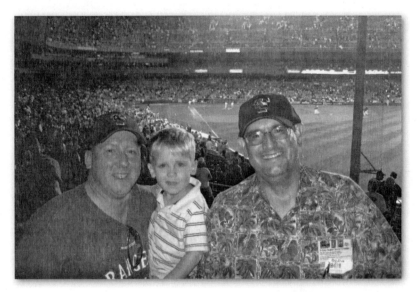

Wishing for T-Bone Miller in Yankee Stadium

Our second Labor Day Family Fun Weekend was another great time. We played the same games and varied our activities to some extent, but for me, it was another celebration of life.

Other than the covenant that I made with Dee Rollins on June 27, 2006, a covenant that I made about four months post-transplant was the most significant of my life with a new heart. I joined the Natatorium where Mary was now swimming and began the process of swimming as exercise for the rest of my life. At first, I just did activity in the water, and then I would swim on my back. I had honestly never learned to swim free style. A young lifeguard agreed to help me learn to swim free style. I took one lesson from her and then was on my own.

Mary and I had planned that if I got a heart transplant, we would go to Mount Rushmore and Yellowstone National Park.

We left in mid-September and had a great time. We came back through central Wyoming and stopped in Rocky Mountain National Park in Colorado. As we crossed eastern Colorado, Mary began to get very seriously ill. She threw-up everywhere: in our hotel room, in the restaurant parking lot, etc. I hoped it would blow over after a good night's sleep. It didn't. I called Mary's physician, Dr. Linda Yeatts, in Denton. She called a prescription that might help to a pharmacy where we were in Goodland, Kansas. Dr. Yeatts was on her way out of town, so when Mary only got sicker, I took her to the emergency room of the small hospital in Goodland. We spent about five hours in the emergency room having X-rays and blood work done. They didn't have a clue of what was causing the problem. We left Goodland late in the afternoon for Dodge City, hoping Mary would be better as we tried to get home. I had to pull to the side of the road for her to throw-up multiple times. We got to Dodge City very late and immediately went to bed. She slept okay. I got up early and looked around at my "Earp" heritage for a few minutes, and then I loaded her up and determined to get her to Denton as soon as possible. Just outside of Cheyenne, Oklahoma, I pulled into a roadside park. Mary hung her head out the door and threw-up over and over. I worried that she would be dehydrated and considered calling 911. I drove into Cheyenne, a small town of about a thousand. There was a small hospital with a one-nurse ER. She quickly took compassion on us and called the doctor. He came quickly, reviewed the blood work, and heard the history of our two-day ordeal; he suspected it might have been food poisoning from some cookies Mary had eaten in Wyoming. He gave her a shot that he felt would enable her to make it the 240 miles to Denton. We made it to Denton and Mary then spent a frustrating four days at Denton Regional Hospital. She was in agony with gut pain, the pain only softened some by a very strong painkillers. The doctors thought it was her severe back issues, somehow manifesting themselves in her abdominal pain. We took her home and she gradually improved over a period of a couple of weeks. We never knew for sure the cause of this difficult time for her.

By November, I had finished the prednisone, the first step in the anti-rejection battle. I had been told that the first year post-transplant was the most critical, and that I needed to make it five years to get to a point where rejection was not as much of an issue. I was just six months post-transplant, but so far so good. I was glad to see that now instead of taking almost sixty pills a day I was down to fewer than forty. Keeping up with the medication was a daunting task. I understood that some people who had transplants didn't make it because they were not careful and precise with their medication. I did not want to make that mistake. But to take the pills from eleven prescriptions, plus vitamins and supplements, at the right time and in the right amount and keep the prescriptions refilled took lots of focus on my part. Long ago, one of the best things that Mary had done for me was to expect me to take care of my own medical issues as much as possible. Others would dote over me; she would say, "Let him learn to do it." I am convinced that Mary's influencing me to take ownership of my own medication issues is a main reason I am alive today.

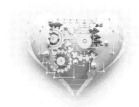

KNEE REPLACEMENT

There was much to be thankful for at Thanksgiving, and we looked forward to the first Christmas with a new heart. In mid-December, I awoke one morning and started to get out of bed. My knee buckled with excruciating pain. There was no preliminary decline, no warning. I could not stand up. The knee replacement that never happened was coming home to roost. My original orthopedic doctor in Denton, Dr. Kristofferson, agreed to see me. He gave me a shot in the knee but held little encouragement that it would last long. He said his medical notes from 1995 noted that both my knees needed replacing. I asked if there was anything that would buy a little time, as I was still only seven months post-transplant. In January he gave me a series of injections over a period of three weeks. He felt it might buy some time, but did not give me a lot of encouragement. I felt I needed to make it until I had been one year post transplant in May. He told me that he did not want to do the knee replacement in Denton. It needed to be done at Baylor, with the heart doctors close. I had consulted with Dr. Kurt Rathjen at Baylor about my knees previously. I scheduled an appointment with him and we agreed on May 18, 2009, as a surgery date. This would be almost exactly one year post-transplant.

I marked one year post-transplant in several ways. One was to attend the annual Baylor heart/lung transplant picnic on a beautiful, sunny Sunday afternoon. Baylor has a significant history of being a regional organ transplantation center. When I had my transplant, I had been given a card that showed that my transplant was number 576 in Baylor organ transplant history. When the heart transplant group photo was taken, there were about twenty of us. The other way that I marked one year post-transplant was to write a letter to the Southwest Transplant alliance that coordinates all the transplants in the southwest USA. I had been told that after one year, I would be allowed to initiate contact and see if the family of the heart donor was open to contact. The letter was the way that was done.

Meanwhile, I got a call from Dr. Rathjen's office and was asked to reschedule the knee replacement surgery to June 15, 2009. The scheduling of my surgery was extremely difficult because of the variety of doctors who needed to be available in case of complications.

Dr. Rathjen and I had agreed that my left knee was the one most badly in need of replacement. He had hoped that I would be able to go home within a week after the surgery. The day of the surgery, I looked at my hospital ID bracelet and noted that this would be my thirtieth hospitalization at Baylor! By now, they should know me when they see me coming! Because of my bad gut problem following the transplant, Mary and I carefully told Dr. Rathjen and everyone else we saw on the day of the surgery that we did not want a recurrence of that. All the doctors and staff seemed to hear what we were saying; in retrospect, they didn't really. The knee replacement was successful and the recovery and physical therapy process began. However, I quickly realized there was something wrong in my gut. No one seemed to believe me. "Oh, everyone feels that way," or "It'll clear up," was the attitude of very busy people who didn't understand how well I knew my own body. In a few days, I was throwing-up literally all over the room. All the physical therapy for my knee immediately went to the backburner. I went NPO and one of the notorious nose-tubes was inserted in the middle of a crisis-filled night. I watched as the dark, ugly bile spewed into the container on the wall. It was identical to the experience the previous year. Dr. Lamont, who had been my doctor in the previous intestinal blockage episode, was called in. I had two CAT scans and nine-teen X-rays over the next few days. He said that I had a bowel obstruction, but he hoped it would clear if we were just patient and waited. It seemed to clear in a few days and thankfully the nose-tube was pulled, and I was allowed to eat soups and Jell-o. Hopefully the blockage had cleared. Then I had the worst throwing-up episode of all. I was embarrassed and frustrated as three nurses had to gown-up and literally clean the whole room. I was approaching two weeks in the hospital. I did not want to think of the possibility of another surgery.

There was no other choice. On Monday night, June 29, Dr. Lamont and his assistant opened up my abdomen and cleared the blockage. They found that my abdominal lining was in shreds. "It looked like Swiss cheese," Dr. Lamont later told me. So, he sewed in a large lining made from pig intestines across my entire abdomen. The surgery took almost three hours, and I went, once again, to Roberts ICU. This three-week hospital stay with its two surgeries was the worst of my thirty hospitalizations at Baylor. Dr. Kuiper came every day to check on me.

On Sunday, July 5, in the midst of a long holiday weekend, I was ready to come home in every way except physically. The holiday weekend meant a short staff and not much physical therapy activity. One of doctor Lamont's assistants came by about the time that Dr. Kuiper did. I asked boldly what the chances of them sending me home were. Without a host of others around to consult, the attitude of these two young, aggressive doctors was, "Why not?" They agreed that Dr. Kuiper would pull all the tubes (I had had to have a PICC line inserted) while the other doctor wrote the orders. Mary arrived thinking she was there to visit, not knowing that I had plotted my escape. Never had I been more relieved to leave a hospital.

Honestly, I was not able to go home, but I believed that if I did not make my escape that day that by the time all the other doctors were back after the holiday weekend, I would have languished at Baylor several more days. I quickly realized that being home was no picnic. Later that night the "nacho kid" patiently pulled me to my feet off the commode. I would not have made it to bed without him. That was the beginning of one of the most difficult parts of my entire journey of life. I did not come back quickly or easily. The two surgeries left me weak and full of doubt whether I would gain my strength. I had a physical therapist come to the house and help me make gradual progress. My lack of energy and will worried Mary. What I needed was a kick in the behind. Rachel delivered that a week later, when our family converged on our house for supper. "You need to get going and get better," she said. "Everyone depends on you, so suck it up and work harder at it." I did.

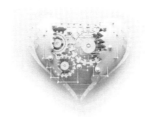

DONOR FAMILY

While I had been at Baylor, Mary had called me from Denton one day after she had gotten the mail. A response had been received from the Southwest Transplant alliance that the donor family was open to hear from me. Now that I was about three weeks into my rehab and beginning to make progress, one afternoon I called the number that I had been given for Calista Aston. She is the widow of the heart donor, James Aston, who was forty-two years old at the time of his death. She is an RN and she and her three children Crystal, Nicholas, and Tabitha, live in Era, Texas, about twenty-five miles from Denton. We talked over the phone and exchanged e-mails. Then we arranged to meet for dinner in Sanger, Texas. Our family bonded with hers at the outset. As she shared their experience, we could see the ways in which God had answered the prayers that we had prayed for them while awaiting the transplant. When we had our third annual Labor Day Family Fun Weekend in a few weeks, Calista, Nicholas, and Tabitha were with us.

We had been confused the night before my transplant after waiting so long with constantly changing schedules. Dr. Kuiper had said the transplant would be rescheduled to the next morning due to the lack of availability of an operating room. We had been around Baylor so many years that we knew there were many operating rooms. The confusion was finally cleared up when we met Calista and her family and they shared their story. Her husband James in a time of distress and discouragement about life had shot himself in the head the Sunday before the transplant on Thursday. He had been careflighted to another hospital in Dallas, and though brain dead, had remained on life support for several days. Those days enabled Calista and her children and their support group from their church to gather in Dallas and spend some final time. Prayers for grace for them, still unknown to us, were answered. That time on life support also provided the opportunity for Calista to make the decision that James' organs would be donated. The operating room availability issue had not been at Baylor, but at the other hospital when James died. In addition to the heart that I received, three other organs were donated.

God takes the most tragic circumstances and brings good from them. Out of this family's tragedy, four other lives received organs and for them, life continued. As a result, I am alive today. It reminded me of the serious conversation that I had had with my granddaughter Tatum about me having a transplant being "sad" because someone else had to die. That is such an enormous emotional and spiritual issue. My doctors had encouraged me to not let the emotions of the situation bother me, saying that the donor would have died any how. The organs being donated in fact brought new life out of that death. I understood more clearly the day I met Calista and her family. We took pictures together and then lingered for a few minutes. Before I left, Calista and her son Nickolas wanted to listen to my chest to hear the heartbeat. I cannot think of a better picture to encourage the donation of organs than having Nickolas stand with his ear next to my chest, listening to the heart beat of his father's heart in me.

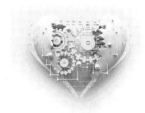

WHAT'S IT LIKE?

As in the days when I lived with an LVAD, I can tell that people around me are curious, but reluctant to ask about my circumstances. Only recently did a young man who knew that I had a heart transplant ask whether I had all kinds of new cravings, as if somehow the transplant had changed me such that I acquired the characteristics of another person. Mary and I have often discussed how the transplant has changed both of us.

I mentioned earlier how I no longer perspire. That and the mysterious spot in my hair are the only visible physical changes. The most welcome change obviously is a regular blood flow in my body. But remember that I didn't just go from my natural heart to a donated heart. I went from a three year existence with an LVAD to the donated heart, which meant leaving behind batteries, dressing changes, vent filters, the constant noise, the vibration of the LVAD inside me, the inability to shower, and the uncertainty if I would live another day.

I have changed in monumental ways emotionally, mentally, and spiritually. When I wake up in the morning, it is not just like any other day of my life. I realize that my life for that new day is a gift. Of course I get hungry, I get angry, I get grumpy, I feel joy, I laugh, and I cry. At the end of some days I have to acknowledge sin that disgusts me - impure thoughts, disrespect for God,

His creatures, and His creation. I confess my sin and ask for His forgiveness. I had previously lived each day with all these "normal" issues, but I had never lived with a sense every new day that life is a gift. It is a gift. I know it. I am humbled by it. Without God's mercy and healing, without a donor heart, there would be no life today. The result is a different way of viewing life. I have a new perspective.

Honestly I used to hold onto life so tightly with my stress and worry and anxiety. Living with life as a gift means holding on so much more loosely. I know that where I am, what I have, and what I am doing in the moment is temporal and will not last. It is not to be grasped, for it cannot and will not last. I live life much more directly in the shadow of eternity. I realize that sometimes I get what I want and sometimes I don't. While I still relish a good discussion of some deep thought after reading a C.S. Lewis insight, I live more simply by the truth from the Forest Gump statement, "life is a like a box of chocolates; you never know what you are going to get." As a transplant patient that is especially true. When I wake up in the morning, I may feel nauseated and in physical malaise. When that happens, Mary gets the transplant book out and we work to see if there are adjustments that need to be made in medications or lifestyle. The next day things may be better, and we never even know why the malaise of the previous day occurred.

I was initially so emotional after I lived, that for a long time I was on an anti-depressant to stabilize my moods. I can still cry at a moments notice, or be grumpy with my grandchildren. I wish afterwards always that I had responded differently. I get tired easily and don't have the stamina to do projects that were once easy.

However, in the midst of these still challenging realities, there is a freedom to live without worry or fear. Small frustrations don't easily sabotage my day. Disappointments and failures don't suck the joy out of life. Aspirations and desire for recognition don't hold a grip on me. People, not things, are a priority. A conversation with a small child, singing fun songs with my grandchildren, slowly watching a sunset, or looking for a rainbow are all the pure joys of life. This is the gift of life. Constantly there are these inner thoughts: life is a gift so I better live well, and "this is really living."

Another question that people are afraid to ask is, "what's it like to lose a son?"

Mary and I often struggle for answers. David's death caused us to want to know more about heaven. Mary was led to a book a few years ago that helped us and inspired us to develop a study on heaven that we have done multiple times. We have many perplexing conversations about prayer. In some cases, we see clear answers. In some, we don't.

Two years ago Mary and I were asked to share at a conference on prayer. We struggled mightily regarding sharing our deepest thoughts and questions. At such times, the common testimony is that God answers prayers. The afternoon before the conference, we were returning from a trip in our car. For several hours we shared back and forth on what we might say at the conference. Finally, Mary blurted out, "I can't do this. I can't stand up with a smile on my face and say that God answers prayers. If He did, David would still be alive." Her stark honesty had returned us to a familiar place in our relationship. We have often been at that place, sharing our perplexity and frustration at the unfairness of it. No matter how many times we go over this, we arrive back at the same place. David died, and we can't change that. That is such a devastating and emotionally draining issue. In spite of our tears and our prayers and our giving our lives as parents to protect him, he still died! How unfair! How awful! We don't understand what God's purpose was in allowing David to die. Those are our honest feelings, but because of our Christian faith, we live by the truth, and not our feelings. We know the truth to be that God loves us and that He loved David. He did have purpose for David's life, but we can't fully see it yet. So, as we always come back to the same place about David, we remind each other of these truths—no matter how contrary to our feelings they seem. We have since sat with others who lost their children, as they grieved and lashed out at the unfairness of life. We inwardly and quietly prayed for them that in the face of their feelings, eventually they would find solid comfort and assurance in God's truths.

What could we say at the conference that was honest and truthful, yet recognized the power and sovereignty of God? We listened at various testimonies at the prayer conference about the special way that God had answered prayer—powerfully and marvelously for the benefit of the situation or persons prayed for. When our turn came, we shared truthfully that we needed especially to pray for those who did not get the outcome they prayed for - that they might be given God's grace to see them through their grief and their anger.

We are aware that when some people are facing life threatening illnesses, our calls or visits leave them uncomfortable. They honestly would rather be hearing from someone whose prayers for healing were answered. But when we embrace someone close who has lost their loved one, we sense that they hug us in a special way, knowing that we have been at the same station of the journey that they are on. Our best encouragement is to give our love, pray for God's grace, and share their loss. We listen to their anger and embrace them in their weeping, for we too have been there.

"Why don't you move on with life?" is a question that we hear people ask. That sounds easy, but it is very, very difficult to do when you lose a child. I still find myself submerged in grief on occasion. But the greatest truth that always comes to me, even in the pit of despair, is that God is the author of life, and if He grants life, I can live it with his help with fervor and meaning. For reasons only He knows, I am alive and David is not–but thankfully David is in heaven. I will be there too, sooner or later. With His help, Mary and I marvel at the complexity and mystery of eternity. We long to see everyone we encounter in this life in heaven. Only then will we see clearly and understand fully.

What's it like to live through hell on earth, year after year? No one has ever asked us this question directly, even though we know they want to. We recognize the value of David's encounter with Don Piper and our common understanding that while Don's book was about heaven, God intended to use it in our life to share his experience of hell on earth. There is real fellowship in common suffering. We now understand by our own experience a scripture that we had often read from Ephesians 3:10: "I want to know Christ, and the power of his resurrection, and the *fellowship of sharing in his sufferings...*" Everyone wants to know the power of his resurrection, but we flinch at the thought of being in the fellowship of those sharing in his sufferings. The sufferings of others bring great perspective. At a critical time in my life in the midst of suffering, I was drawn to read *When God Weeps* by Joni Eareckson Tada. I was humbled and awed as I read her reflections of her own sufferings of living almost forty years as a quadriplegic in a wheel chair. Then as she detailed the excruciating pain and sufferings of others, I recognized that my sufferings paled in comparison. No matter the magnitude of our common sufferings, there is great comfort and help in fellowship. Mary and I see that is the reason for our story. We have now been through nine years of what some would say is the worst life has to offer. What life lessons have we learned?

First, the truth that because we are believers, God is with us in the suffering. He knows where we are and He loves us. Yet in the midst of those terrible times, we often cannot see the evidence of this in our circumstances. We wonder where God is, and why He has allowed us to be in such a wasteland. Thus, we have to walk by faith and not by sight.

Next, we learned an analogy that eternally changed our perspective. It is the analogy of the two rails. Our tendency is to see life as a series of good days and bad days and always seek for that time when there will only be good days. However, the truth from the analogy is that there are always two parallel rails in life–one good and one bad—running along side each other. We will always have some good and we will always have some bad. Life will never be only good or only bad. Accepting that truth, the focus in the bad rail times is to look for the good. We have learned in the worst times, to look for good. There are even moments of humor in the worst times of life.

Finally, we have learned that life is really not about what happens to us, but how we respond to what happens to us. That attitude in the midst of the worst of times has enabled us to keep on going. We believe sharing these thoughts in this book is the culmination of that. We pray for you and encourage you to recognize that although you do not have a choice about what happens to you, you do have a choice about how you respond. We invite you into the fellowship of those who suffer, but recognize that it is a momentary thing in the great perspective of eternity.

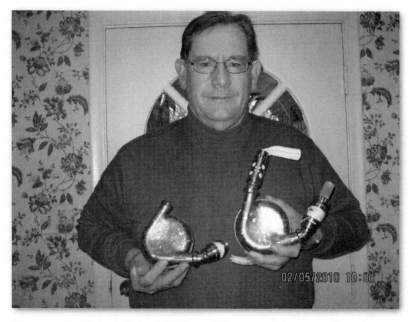

Governor holding the two LVADs and living with his transplanted heart

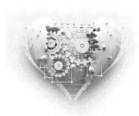

EPILOGUE

Life with purpose continues. I recently sat at Rose Lawn Cemetery at our family plot where our son David is buried. I glanced just a few feet to the right where my "space" is. Sooner or later, I will die and be buried in that place. Until then, I resolve to live well, remembering the three-fold mandate that God gave me when He preserved my life in 2005. *Be a role model for your family.* I pray every day this is so. We now have a tradition that came from this mandate—the Labor Day Family Fun Weekend. May my grandchildren and the generations that follow them be blessed that God allowed me to live. *Care for the poor and downtrodden.* The recent earthquake in Haiti reminded me once again how important the orphans and poor are. I am alive for this work. My church will make a mission trip to Haiti this year. I continue to encourage my dear friend in Haiti, Jacob Bernard. He and Claudette are alive today, miraculously, as are many orphans under their care. I serve on the Board of Directors of Mission Possible Foundation, which ministers to the poor and to the street children in Albania, Bulgaria, and Russia. Our church will make a mission trip to Russia in 2011. *Write a book.* Here it is, finally, all by God's grace.

So much for "the Governor." What about you? Since you chose to read the book, I have one question, which can be worded in different ways: "Are you living well?" Or, as my brother-in-law, Jack would say, "Are you really living?" I remember the words of Jesus of Nazareth, who said, "I have come that you might have life, and have it to the full." Do you have life to the full?

I hope that you get the truth from this book that living well, really living, life to the full, is not about being comfortable or carefree. It is about living with passion to make a difference in the lives of others, in spite of trouble or circumstances. It is about being in the game, and suffering the injuries, the pain, and the setbacks. Living well is not about being a spectator in the grandstands, watching others wage the battles. It is about getting into the arena, living intentionally, with gritty determination. One of my favorite quotations is from a speech delivered by Theodore Roosevelt in 1910. In this speech he says, "The credit belongs to the man who is actually *in the arena*, whose face is marred by dust and sweat and blood, who strives valiantly, who errs, who comes short again and again, because there is no effort without error and shortcoming, but who does actually strive to do the deeds, who knows great enthusiasms, the great devotions, who spends himself in a worthy cause, who, at the best, knows in the end the triumph of high achievement, and who at the worst, if he fails, at least fails while daring greatly, so that his place shall never be with those cold and timid souls who neither know victory nor defeat."

Are you *in the arena?*

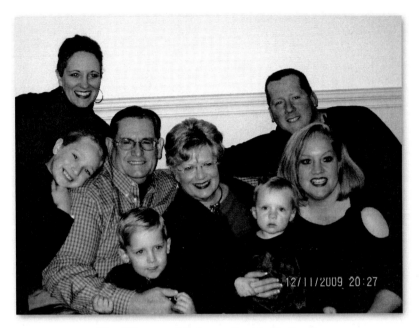

The "Governor" living well with his family